MEDICAL INNOVATION AT THE CROSSROADS

VOLUME V

Sources of Medical Technology:
Universities and Industry

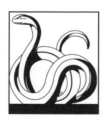

Nathan Rosenberg, Annetine C. Gelijns, and Holly Dawkins, Editors

Committee on Technological Innovation in Medicine

INSTITUTE OF MEDICINE

NATIONAL ACADEMY PRESS
Washington, D.C.   1995

NATIONAL ACADEMY PRESS • 2101 Constitution Avenue, N.W. • Washington, D.C. 20418

The Institute of Medicine was chartered in 1970 by the National Academy of Sciences to enlist distinguished members of the appropriate professions in the examination of policy matters pertaining to the health of the public. In this the Institute acts under both the Academy's 1863 congressional charter responsibility to be an advisor to the federal government and its own initiative in identifying issues of medical care, research, and education. Dr. Kenneth I. Shine is president of the Institute of Medicine.

The Committee on Technological Innovation in Medicine was established in 1988 by the Institute of Medicine to design a series of workshops that would (a) provide more fundamental knowledge of the process by which biomedical research findings are translated into clinical practice and (b) address opportunities for improving the rationality and efficiency of the process. This volume consists of the proceedings of the fifth workshop in the series, "The University-Industry Interface and Medical Innovation," held in Stanford, California, on February 21–23, 1993. This workshop and its proceedings were supported by the Howard Hughes Medical Institute and Pfizer. The opinions and conclusions expressed here are those of the authors and do not necessarily represent the views of the National Academy of Sciences, any of its constituent parts, or the organizations providing support.

Library of Congress Cataloging-in-Publication Data

Sources of medical technology : universities and industry / Annetine
    C. Gelijns and Nathan Rosenberg, editors ; Committee on
    Technological Innovation in Medicine, Institute of Medicine.
        p.   cm. — (Medical innovation at the crossroads ; v. 5)
      Includes bibliographical references and index.
      ISBN 0-309-05189-4
      1. Medical innovations. 2. Medicine—Research. I. Gelijns,
    Annetine. II. Rosenberg, Nathan. III. Institute of Medicine
    (U.S.). Committee on Technological Innovation in Medicine.
    IV. Series.
      [DNLM: 1. Diffusion of Innovation. 2. Technology, Medical.
    3. Research Support—United States. W1 ME342f v. 5 1994 / W 20.5
    S724 1994]
    RA418.5.M4S68   1994
610'.72—dc20
DNLM/DLC
for Library of Congress   94-43303
                                                      CIP

Printed in the United States of America

The serpent has been a symbol of long life, healing, and knowledge among almost all cultures and religions since the beginning of recorded history. The image adopted as a logotype by the Institute of Medicine is based on a relief carving from ancient Greece, now held at the Staatlichemuseen in Berlin.

Committee on Technological Innovation in Medicine

Acknowledgments

The Committee on Technological Innovation in Medicine wishes to acknowledge and thank the many individuals and organizations who contributed their time, knowledge, and energy to the production of this volume. First and foremost, the committee thanks the authors of the chapters in this book; early drafts of these chapters were originally presented at the Institute of Medicine (IOM) workshop entitled "The University-Industry Interface" (see Appendix A for the agenda of this meeting) but much thought and effort went into their further development. The committee also expresses its gratitude to the meeting moderators, discussants, and participants. Great appreciation is also due to Dana O'Neil, who worked hard to coordinate the on-site workshop logistics, and Kenneth Melmon and Nathan Rosenberg, the "local" committee members, on whom we imposed with various demands, of varied urgency, both before and during the workshop.

The intellectual origins of this volume are found in the interests of Kenneth Melmon and Nathan Rosenberg in examining the interdisciplinary and interinstitutional aspects of medical innovation, to whom the committee is deeply indebted. The committee also expresses its gratitude to Annetine C. Gelijns, who, as the past program director, dedicated much time, thought, and energy to developing and refining the volume's focus. Others, however, were also critical: Kathleen N. Lohr, director of the Division of Health Care Services; Enriqueta Bond, the IOM's executive director until mid-1994; Karl D. Yordy, previous director of the Division; and the current and past IOM Presidents Kenneth I. Shine and

Samuel O. Thier all spring to mind for their generous and steady support of the program.

Among the IOM project staff who worked on this volume, the committee particularly recognizes Holly Dawkins, whose commitment and contributions to the series since its inception have been a vital factor in its production, and Helen Rogers, recognized for her superb management of the workshop logistics and her skilled support of the committee's work. Other staff members to be thanked are Don Tiller, who added the administrative tasks of this volume to his already heaped pile of tasks and put in weekend hours to assure its timely delivery to the press; Mike Edington, honored as the Institute of Medicine's managing editor, who swept away or diminished the various obstacles in the staffs' path; Nina Spruill, who has managed the complicated financial aspects of *Medical Innovation at the Crossroads* with good will and extraordinary ability for nigh on five years; and Susan Knasiak and Jay Ball, both of whom provided able and critical secretarial assistance during production of this book.

The committee thanks various organizations for their financial support of the workshop and of the *Medical Innovation at the Crossroads* series. This volume would not exist without the continued support of the Howard Hughes Medical Institute and Pfizer.

In closing, the committee recognizes that today's rapid changes in the financing and delivery of U.S. health care may well have a significant effect on the incentives for universities and industrial firms to generate new medical technologies. This volume examines the changing roles and interactions of these two critical participants in technological change. It is this committee's hope that this book provides a starting point for further research on these critical, but often neglected, institutional interactions in the innovation process.

Gerald D. Laubach
Chair
Committee on Technological
Innovation in Medicine

Contents

List of Tables and Figures

TABLES

FIGURES

ix

List of Abbreviations

ACP	American College of Physicians
ACMI	American Cystoscope Makers, Inc.
AIRs	Academy Industry Relations
AO	American Optical
AQ	acoustic quantification
beta-gal	beta-galactosidase
CCD	charge couple device
cDNA	complementary deoxyribonucleic acid
CO_2	carbon dioxide
CRADAs	cooperative research and development agreements
CSFs	colony stimulating factors
CT	computerized tomography
DHSS	British Department of Health
DOA	Department of Agriculture
ENT	ear, nose, and throat
EPO	erithropoietin
ERCP	endoscopic retrograde cholangiopancreatography
FDA	Food and Drug Administration
GI	gastrointestinal
HCFA	Health Care Financing Administration
HIMA	Health Industry Manufacturers Association
HP	Hewlett-Packard
HPLC	high-performance liquid chromatography
IBA	Industrial Biotechnology Association
IEEE	Institute of Electronics and Electrical Engineers

JSEP	Joint Services Electronics Program
LASER	light amplification by stimulated emission of radiation
MIS	minimally invasive surgery
MIT	Massachusetts Institute of Technology
MRC	Medical Research Council
MRI	magnetic resonance imaging
mRNA	messenger ribonucleic acid
NBFs	new biotechnology firms
ND3	deuterated ammonia
Nd:YAG	neodymium-doped yttrium-aluminum-garnet
NEN	New England Nuclear
NIH	National Institutes of Health
NIST	National Institute of Standards and Technology
NSF	National Science Foundation
NTIS	National Technical Information Service
OSTP	Office of Science and Technology Policy
PET	positron emission tomography
PPS	Prospective Payment System
R&D	research and development
RAC	Recombinant DNA Advisory Committee
rDNA	recombinant deoxyribonucleic acid
SBA	Small Business Administration
SPECT	single photon emission computerized tomography
Tc	technetium-99
TC	tissue characterization
TEE	transesophageal echocardiography
t-PA	tissue plasminogen activator
TRG	technical research group
UCSF	University of California, San Francisco

Sources of Medical Technology: Universities and Industry

PART I

Setting the Stage

1

The Changing Nature of Medical Technology Development

ANNETINE C. GELIJNS AND NATHAN ROSENBERG

It is axiomatic in recent discussions of health care in the United States that its quality and cost have been transformed almost beyond recognition in the years since the end of World War II. A fundamental component of that transformation has been a rapid rate of technological change that has led to the insertion into the health care system of a range of new diagnostic and therapeutic technologies that had no real antecedent in prewar years. The recognition that medical technology is a critical element in the quality as well as the cost of health care has renewed interest in the factors shaping technological change or innovation in medicine. At a more general level, one can observe that medical innovation is stimulated by advances in scientific and engineering knowledge, on the one hand, and by the potential demand for health-improving technology, on the other. The health care reform debate, however, has been dominated by a preoccupation with *demand*-side factors. In particular, discussions have focused on how changes in demand-side incentives, as precipitated, for instance, by the introduction of global budgets, higher insurance co-payments, and the like, might reduce the cost-ineffective use of existing medical interventions and alter the direction of medical innovation toward the development of cost-reducing technologies. By comparison, the conditions governing the *supply* of new medical technologies, and their particular characteristics, have been relatively neglected. It is this lacuna that the present volume attempts to address.

At the outset, we need to recognize that policy discussions of technological change have often been impoverished by the notion that innovation is a more or less homogeneous activity, as is implied by the "linear model." The truth, of course, is that innovation is not one thing; it is many things. The processes by

3

which new technologies are generated differ enormously from one sector of the economy to another. Nothing is more likely to muddy the waters of understanding, and therefore muddy the policymaking process as well, than the notion that we are dealing with a uniform set of relationships when we move from one sector of the economy to the next, carrying with us the assumption that "one size fits all." The beginning of wisdom is the recognition of the extreme diversity of background conditions underlying the innovation process. Arrangements that may work well in semiconductors or the aircraft industry may not work well at all in pharmaceuticals. Indeed, what has worked well in pharmaceuticals may not work at all in the newly emerging biotechnology sector. Moreover, if we consider new clinical procedures or medical devices, the conditions for successful innovation are probably very different from other subsectors of the medical technology realm. Even within these subsectors, there is considerable diversity in this respect. Consider, for example, medical devices. Medical devices encompass a heterogeneous group of products, ranging from low tech, inexpensive devices such as tongue depressors and disposable needles, to sophisticated and expensive modalities such as lithotripters and magnetic resonance imaging (MRI) machines. Obviously, the research required for the invention of, for example, disposable needles is quite different from that required for the invention of the computerized tomography (CT) scanner; the heterogeneity in products, and their research and development (R&D) strategies, is reflected in the manufacturers that produce these products.

If we focus on the conditions governing the supply of new medical technologies, two characteristics emerge that merit specific attention in this respect. First, evidence suggests that medical innovation is becoming increasingly dependent on interdisciplinary research.[1] That is, the successful development of a particular technology frequently requires close cooperation among a growing number of individuals with diverse but relevant professional backgrounds. In the case of pharmaceuticals and biologicals, for example, the development of a drug may require cooperation among organic chemists, molecular biologists, immunologists, material scientists, toxicologists, chemical engineers, clinicians, and so on. In the case of medical devices, the interdisciplinary nature of innovation appears even more obvious. The development of devices generally depends on the transfer of scientific and technological advances outside of medicine (e.g., in physics, engineering, and their relevant subfields, such as micro-electronics, materials science, optics, etc.) into medicine. It thus requires the interaction of physicists

---

[1] An interesting indication that this is the case can be found in the recent Food and Drug Administration (FDA) guidelines on "combination products." These guidelines were issued because the FDA's traditional division of products into drugs, biologicals, and devices is becoming problematic as an increasing number of products are combinations of drugs, devices, or biologicals—for example, hormone-releasing intrauterine devices.

and engineers with medical specialists. Moreover, medical innovation may require the involvement of a variety of medical specialties. For example, the evolution of cardiopulmonary bypass was dependent upon a range of professions, including, among others, cardiac surgeons, cardiologists, physiologists, anesthesiologists, and hematologists.

Second, innovation requires not only the crossing of disciplinary boundaries, but it also increasingly involves the crossing of institutional boundaries. In fact, medical innovation depends heavily on interactions between universities, particularly academic medical centers, and industrial firms. Over the past decade, the number and diversity of these university-industry interactions have greatly increased (Blumenthal, 1994).

A review of the literature reveals that there is little insight into how these characteristics affect the efficiency with which research findings are translated into clinical practice. The objective of the present volume therefore is to examine how the interdisciplinary and interinstitutional nature of current medical R&D shapes the rate and direction of medical innovation. In doing so, it focuses particularly on the medical device and biotechnology sector.

ORGANIZATION OF THE PRESENT VOLUME

This volume starts out with a discussion of the increase in public and private spending on medical R&D in the United States. As Bond and Glynn (chapter 2) observe, the decades following World War II have been characterized by an impressive growth in federal funding for biomedical research and medical education. This investment vastly strengthened the position of academic medical centers and stimulated the education of a growing cadre of specialists and subspecialists—defining, and redefining, disciplinary boundaries within medicine. Moreover, in recent years, the government has begun more actively to encourage universities to work with manufacturers to stimulate the transfer of their research findings into medical practice. These efforts have led to a marked increase in university-industry interactions.

The core of the volume then examines how the interdisciplinary and interinstitutional nature of medical R&D has shaped the rate and direction of innovation in several major areas of medical intervention (viz., lasers, minimally invasive surgery, cochlear implants, cardiovascular diagnostics, the development of synthetic insulin, and biotechnology agents in general). These analyses generally take a historical approach to the subject. Innovation, by definition, is not only a process that occurs over time; it is, at bottom, a learning process. Research and development activities are conducted in an environment of limited or, at the least, insufficient information. At the outset, the uncertainty level is high. The learning process of innovation is one in which information is accumulated and uncertainties reduced, commonly over the course of extended time periods. Therefore, if we want to explain why a particular innovation occurred when it did, it is misleading to refer to the time that elapsed between a scientific breakthrough and an eventual application as a "lag" (Rosenberg, 1982, particularly chapter 3). Galileo was not the inventor of the pendulum clock, even though he did indeed formulate the scientific principles that govern the behavior of the pendulum clock. Similarly, the basic science underlying light transmission was developed by Christiaan Huygens in the seventeenth century, but it would be preposterous to regard him as the inventor of fiber optics. Huygens's scientific breakthrough, a formidable intellectual advance, tells us nothing about why optical fibers were introduced into endoscopy in the 1950s and 1960s rather than the 1850s and 1860s. Other factors need to be invoked to provide the explanation. Those factors would include drastic improvements in the quality, and manufacturing, of optical glass, as well as essential activities at the levels of applied physics and engineering (see Gelijns and Rosenberg, chapter 4, this volume).

The nonhistorical view of innovation, which "knows how the story ends," continually ignores the uncertainties that prevailed at an earlier date, and assumes that important information was already available long before it was in fact acquired, that is, learned (Rosenberg, 1994b). This is partly because most information, once it has been acquired, appears "obvious." The heliocentric view of the universe is, to us, obvious, but it required many centuries of patient observation and cogitation, as well as the availability of more sophisticated instrumentation, before it became obvious. By contrast, the historical approach—by asking about the innovators "what did they know and when did they know it?"—provides information that is indispensable to a full appreciation of the complexity, the creativity, and the time-consuming nature of the innovation process.

Following the analyses of particular areas of medical innovation in chapters 3 through 8, the volume then provides two perspectives on the management of interdisciplinary and interinstitutional R&D. Laubach (chapter 9) discusses how today's rapidly changing health care environment affects the developer-user interface, and the particular challenges this raises for industrial R&D management. Nelson (chapter 10) briefly examines the intertwining of science and technology in medicine. He raises fundamental questions about what is public and what is private in medicine, and what should be patentable and what should not be patentable in this sector. How we address these questions will have profound implications for the transfer of research findings from academia to industry, as well as for the ease of information exchange within the medical profession.

In the remainder of this introductory chapter, we will address some of the findings of the present volume, and highlight the needs for future research in this area.

IMPORTANCE OF UNIVERSITY-INDUSTRY INTERACTIONS

Medical innovation is a particularly interesting area for examining university-industry interactions in the development and commercialization of technology. Why is this so? One reason is that innovation in this sector provides a rich set of interactions that appear to transcend what might be regarded as the "normal" division of labor between academia and industrial firms.[2] Of course, medical schools are involved in basic biomedical research, and the fruits of their efforts may contribute to the development of new technologies by industrial laboratories. The discovery of recombinant deoxyribonucleic acid (DNA) technology by Boyer and Cohen at the University of California, San Francisco, and Stanford University, for example, directly encouraged the industrial development of such biologicals as human insulin, the growth hormones, and tissue plasminogen activator (see Stern, chapter 7). Medical device innovation, by contrast, does not depend nearly as heavily on the exploitation of basic scientific and technological capabilities generated "upstream" within medical schools as does the pharmaceutical or the emerging biotechnology sector. Instead, it relies heavily on the transfer of technological capabilities already generated outside of the medical sector—and indeed more commonly generated in the industrial world rather than the academic world.

Consider, for example, the lithotripter. The concept of using shock waves for medical purposes emerged out of research at the German aircraft manufacturer Dornier, where physicists were investigating the causes of pitting seen on the surface of spacecraft and supersonic airplanes (Gelijns, 1991). They found that a craft's collision with micrometeorites or raindrops at very high speeds created shock waves that had a destructive effect on surface structures. They also accidentally discovered that such shock waves could travel through the human body without harming tissue, but that brittle materials in the body were destroyed. These findings led Dornier, in collaboration with urologists at the University of Munich, to develop the first lithotripter for the treatment of kidney stones.

We have deliberately cited an instance of a major new medical technology that had its origin in the aircraft industry in order to highlight how the medical device sector differs from pharmaceuticals and biotechnology. The general point is that this sector looks far outside the realm of biomedical research for new technological capabilities. If one were to look only at the most important contributions to diagnostic technology, one would find that the CT scanner drew heavily on advances in computers and mathematics, ultrasound had its origins in submarine warfare, and MRI originated in the work of experimental physicists exploring the structure of the atom. Thus, medical device innovation is not only inherently interdisciplinary but also outward-looking by nature, and depends on the transfer into medicine of advances in such diverse fields as electronics, optics, computers, and the material sciences (see Figure 1-1).

Whereas, in the context of medical device innovation, medical schools may

---

[2]For a related discussion of the role played by universities in the development of scientific instruments, see "Scientific instrumentation and university research," chapter 13 in Rosenberg, 1994a.

not have been the dominant source of basic scientific and technological knowledge, they do nevertheless play a major and multifaceted role in the development of new medical devices (the "D" of R&D). In academic medical centers, it has been the clinicians rather than basic medical researchers who have most commonly been crucial to the invention of medical devices. They not only identify the clinical need for a new device or for improvements in existing devices but, because of their role as eventual users, they may also be the innovators and builders of the original prototype. Von Hippel and Finkelstein (1979), for example, underlined the importance of these users with regard to the invention of the automated clinical chemical analyzer. The chapters in this volume on endoscopes and cochlear implants (chapters 4 and 5) present similar findings. An exception may be found in the case of nuclear cardiology and echocardiography, where the complexity and multitude of engineering skills required for prototype development were not easily carried out in a clinical research setting (see Finkelstein, Neels, and Bell, chapter 6).

In addition, this volume reveals that in certain cases clinicians may be involved in the manufacturing process. For example, the chapter on minimally invasive surgery (chapter 4) illustrates that the academic/medical community not only developed the first prototype of a flexible gastroenterological endoscope, but that they were also instrumental in teaching the industrial firm how to solve some complicated manufacturing problems—the making of the fiber-optic bundles. This is, to say the least, a drastic departure from what might be regarded as the "normal" division of labor between academics and private industry.

Finally, the academic medical profession plays a critical role during the clinical development, and refinement, process of new medical technology. The medical profession is instrumental and indispensable in evaluating the clinical potential of new devices and drugs during the premarketing development period. As might be expected, feedback at this point may lead to important changes in the design of these products. The development process does *not*, however, end with the more widespread introduction of a new product into practice. New technologies, in medicine as elsewhere, typically enter the world in a primitive condition. In fact, as we will see, important shortcomings may emerge only after extensive use in practice. Once identified, such shortcomings provide the basis for further modification and improvement. This is illustrated by the history of oral contraceptives. The widespread introduction of the first oral contraceptives into clinical practice during the early 1960s confirmed their high degree of effectiveness, but also revealed that their use increased the risk for thromboembolic disorders. The suspicion, based upon subsequent research, that estrogen might be responsible for such circulatory diseases stimulated manufacturers to reduce estrogen levels and develop low-dose pills, which subsequently led to a dramatic decline in side effects (Gelijns and Rosenberg, 1994). Thus, actual adoption constitutes only the beginning of an often prolonged process in which important redesigning takes place, exploiting the feedback of new information generated by

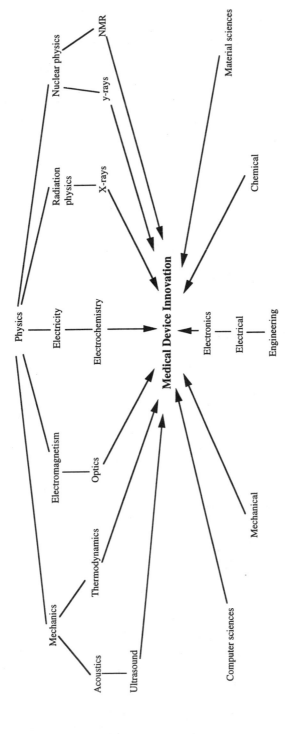

FIGURE 1-1 Example of the interdisciplinary foundations of innovation. SOURCE: Reiser and Anbar, 1984.

users. This incremental improvement process occurs not only in industrial laboratories, but also within clinical practice itself. For example, after new medical devices and biologicals are introduced into clinical practice, the medical profession often discovers entirely new indications of use. A case in point is the laser (see Spetz, chapter 3). Originally introduced for use in ophthalmology and dermatology, it is now being used for a wide variety of indications in oncology, thoracic surgery, and gynecology—to name but a few. Thus, there is an important feedback loop by which improvements, as well as new indications, are extracted from the accumulation of clinical experience with novel instruments and biologicals.

In medicine, therefore, it is of the utmost importance for industrial firms to create close interactions with clinicians, often in academic medical centers. At the same time, clinicians have strong incentives to be involved in the development of new technologies. New technologies, of course, are vital for improving clinical practice. In addition, their use may confer prestige and provide professional recognition in the form of publications. Moreover, the internal dynamics of the medical profession—and the hierarchical scientific status of different subspecialties—is such that innovation is a means for enhancing the professional status of particular medical disciplines. Thus, the intertwining of interests of academic medical specialists and segments of the manufacturing industry tends to encourage an ongoing process of innovation. Blume has argued that we should regard this innovation process as taking place not in a market (in which buyers' and sellers' interests are assumed to be opposed), but rather in an interorganizational field (Blume, 1992).

An extremely interesting finding has been the variety of ways in which these university-industry interactions are accomplished, and indeed the extent to which the organization of activities at the university-industry interface has recently been changing in order to accommodate the needs of the innovation process. Traditionally, interorganizational links have hinged strongly on the movement of personnel between academic and industrial settings, which can range from the hiring of graduate students by industrial firms to consultancy agreements with faculty (Klein, 1990; see also chapter 9, this volume). Nowadays these arrangements are still critically important, but new ways of crossing disciplinary and organizational boundaries are becoming apparent. In the medical device sector, for example, the composition of the industrial R&D team is undergoing significant change in that clinicians are being added to these teams. At the same time, product design engineers, as well as marketing specialists, are receiving more clinical training and are spending more time in academic medical centers.

Another indicator of university-industry interactions can be found in the number, and growth, of licensing agreements. The Boyer-Cohen discovery, for example, provided Stanford with a very profitable patent (chapter 9). Over the past decade, the number of patents that universities have filed in the medical sciences has grown markedly, as well as the number of licensing agreements with industrial firms. Another mechanism for university-industry interactions can be found in research contracts and research agreements. A 12-year, $40 million research agreement, for instance, was recently signed between Harvard Medical School and the Monsanto Company for the development of new interventions for managing cancer (Atkinson, 1994). Such large-scale research agreements are rather unusual. A more common practice these days is that faculty members, and sometimes their parent universities, become involved in the formation of new, start-up companies.

In this respect, small firms can be regarded as transfer mechanisms between traditional university and industrial settings. Small and large companies may play very different roles in the innovation process. In the medical device sector, for example, it has been suggested that small companies—with some notable exceptions—tend to produce the majority of innovations in the early stages of developing a new class of devices, whereas large companies may be more prominent at later stages in the development process (Gelijns and Rosenberg, 1994). Differences in the primary function of small and large device firms, however, should not conceal the complex patterns of relationships that have emerged between the two. Large firms may sponsor research in small firms, often with the intent of acquiring them if their technologies are promising or successful. Furthermore, because recent changes in U.S. payment and regulatory policies have made venture capital funding more difficult, many small firms are seeking alliances with large firms to engage in joint product development, clinical testing, manufacturing, and marketing. Arora and Gambardella (chapter 8) discuss the division of innovative labor in the biotechnology sector and the changing patterns of collaborative alliances between universities, new biotechnology firms, and large pharmaceutical firms.

INTERDISCIPLINARY NATURE OF MEDICAL R&D

We have emphasized the importance of crossing organizational boundaries in the innovation process. In our discussion so far, we have had in mind enterprises such as university research conducted within well-defined academic disciplines on the one hand, and research conducted by industrial firms, large or small, on the other. But there are other boundaries—within these institutions—that may impede the interdisciplinary cooperation and communication necessary for much of today's medical innovation.

In industrial settings, product-related R&D is inevitably interdisciplinary in nature and raises no special challenge to the values and priorities of the organization. Industrial firms are, however, organized into various departments, such as research, product development, manufacturing, and marketing. Management problems have been noted regarding communication and collaboration across these functional activities. For example, Humphrey and Schwartz, at the inaugural meeting of the American Institute for Medical and Biological Engineering in

1992, observed that failure to integrate engineering and manufacturing know-how into the development process of biotechnology drugs prior to phase III clinical trials had locked many final bioprocess designs into nonoptimal processes that did not use leading-edge technology (Humphrey, 1992; Schwartz, 1992).

In the case of academic settings, interdisciplinary R&D may raise some management issues similar to those confronting industrial R&D. Moreover, it may also challenge the basic values and culture of the organization, especially with regard to the pursuit of practical applications of new findings, professional reward structures, and pathways to career advancement. There is little doubt that the organization of the scientific enterprise into disciplines and academic departments has played a major role in the historic success of universities in contributing to the growth of knowledge. Nevertheless, health care problems do not always fall neatly within the boundaries of particular academic disciplines and departments.

Cochlear implants, for example, are essentially interdisciplinary in nature. This has meant that a complex network of different medical specialties were involved in its development. In chapter 5, Blume shows how different patterns of collaboration on cochlear implants evolved, and how these various groups differed considerably in their R&D strategies. In particular, a distinction can be drawn between the more "therapeutically" and the more "experimentally" oriented groups. The therapeutically oriented groups tended to move faster from animal testing to the clinic and collaborated more intensively with industrial firms, whereas the experimental groups entered more slowly into licensing agreements. Blume suggests that the interdisciplinary nature of cochlear implants meant that assembling the necessary skills and competences, securing agreement as to how the value of this new intervention was to be assessed, and establishing what kind of industrial expertise provided commercial advantage was more problematic than in the case of, for example, diagnostic imaging, which is much less interdisciplinary in nature.

The laser and endoscopy chapters (chapters 3 and 4) tell similar stories. The transfer of laparoscopy from gynecology to general surgery, for example, appears to have taken an unnecessarily long time. The authors conclude that "the existing disciplinary boundaries *internal* to medicine itself may have constituted an even more serious obstacle to innovation than those external to medicine. Put somewhat differently, the most difficult barriers that needed to be crossed were not between medicine and industry, but barriers within medicine itself (p. 93)." Medical schools and university teaching hospitals are increasingly recognizing that, to realize the potential of future medical innovation, they may need to build more sturdy bridges between traditional disciplines.

SOME CONCLUDING OBSERVATIONS

The chapters in this volume have, taken together, opened up a number of windows onto a complex and uneven terrain where new medical technologies have emerged. But the individual studies also emphasize that acquiring these technologies is not so much like geographic discovery, where one identifies the features of a terrain that has already been shaped by natural forces; rather, it is more like a creative synthesis, in which elements are taken from very different contexts and then combined in a unique way to achieve some specific improvement in medical care.

Medical device innovation appears to differ considerably from innovation in the realm of pharmacology and biotechnology. Although pharmaceutical and biotechnology innovation also draw upon a number of disciplinary specialties, medical device innovation relies much more heavily upon a systematic intellectual trespassing across well-established disciplinary boundaries. Device innovation, as our studies show, not only draws upon a number of disciplines. It also commonly draws upon technological capabilities that have already been developed elsewhere to serve very different human purposes (e.g., lasers, optical fibers, ultrasound, computers), and it reconfigures and reshapes them to serve very different—that is, medical—purposes.

Future research into the determinants of technological change in medicine must probe more deeply, not only into the problems of communications across disciplinary boundaries (including, increasingly, across the boundaries among medical subspecialties). It also needs to examine the conditions for more effective cooperation across institutional boundaries, including, importantly, the impact of federal regulation upon innovation. In considerable measure, this volume identifies those boundaries as lying at the interface between universities and industry. But, in a larger sense, that interface also corresponds to the boundary between the public and private sectors, between sectors that differ drastically in their sources of finance, their incentives, their responsibilities, and their priorities. These studies also suggest that these boundaries have not been rigid but have been redrawn and reshaped, at least occasionally and in certain specific locations. Moreover, as Laubach's chapter suggests, the recent proposals for health reform on the one hand, and the ongoing transformation of the health care delivery system on the other, are also rapidly transforming the environment within which medical innovation must take place. How these transformations are likely to affect both the rate and the direction of medical innovation needs to become a central concern of both the research community and the policymaker.

REFERENCES

Atkinson, S. H. 1994. University-affiliated venture capital funds. *Health Affairs* 13:159–175.

Blume, S. S. 1992. *Insight and Industry: On the Dynamics of Technological Change.* Cambridge, Mass.: Massachusetts Institute of Technology Press.

Blumenthal, D. 1994. Growing pains for new academic/industry relationships. *Health Affairs* 13:176–193.

Gelijns, A. C. 1991. *Innovation in Clinical Practice: The Dynamics of Medical Technology Development.* Washington, D.C.: National Academy Press.

Gelijns, A. C., and Rosenberg, N. 1994. The dynamics of technological change in medicine. *Health Affairs* 13:28–46.

Humphrey, A. 1992. Challenges to biotechnology in meeting America's future health needs. Presentation at the inaugural meeting of the American Institute of Medical and Biological Engineering, Washington, D.C.

Klein, J. T. 1990. Innovation and change in organizational relationships: Interdisciplinary contexts. *R&D Management* 20:97–102.

Reiser, S. J., and Anbar, M. eds. 1984. *Machine at the Bedside: Strategies for Using Technology in Patient Care.* New York, N.Y.: Cambridge University Press.

Rosenberg, N. 1982. *Inside the Black Box.* New York, N.Y.: Cambridge University Press.

Rosenberg, N. 1994a. *Exploring the Black Box.* New York, N.Y.: Cambridge University Press.

Rosenberg, N. 1994b. Uncertainty and technical change. Unpublished manuscript. Palo Alto, Calif.: Stanford University.

Schwartz, J. 1992. The production of protein pharmaceuticals: Past achievements and future challenges. Presentation at the inaugural meeting of the American Institute of Medical and Biological Engineering, Washington, D.C.

von Hippel, E., and Finkelstein, S. 1979. Analysis of innovation in automated clinical chemistry analyzers. *Science and Public Policy* 6:24–37.

2

Recent Trends in Support for Biomedical Research and Development

ENRIQUETA C. BOND AND SIMON GLYNN

The case studies found in the present volume of the series *Medical Innovation at the Crossroads* explore the role of interdisciplinary and interinstitutional research and development (R&D) in the evolution of modern medical devices and biotechnology drugs. To provide some background for such analysis, this chapter will describe the major sources of financing for biomedical R&D, updating in some respects two useful earlier analyses by Ginzberg and Dutka (1989) and the Institute of Medicine (IOM; 1990). This chapter will also describe recent initiatives to encourage technology transfer by strengthening collaborations between government, industry, and academia. As noted by Weisbrod (1994), a complicated set of financial incentives—such as direct support of R&D in combination with the enormous expansion of health care insurance that has paid for the adoption of technologies—operate to foster technological innovation. As we will see below, both government and industry have substantially increased their investments in R&D but the relative amounts and kinds of investment of the two sectors are changing. Constraints on the federal budget are slowing increases in R&D support by the federal government and leading Congress to demand more evidence of health "payoffs" from these investments.

BIOMEDICAL RESEARCH AND DEVELOPMENT FUNDERS

Total national funding for biomedical R&D exceeded $30 billion in 1993 (U.S. Department of Health and Human Services, 1993). Of this, spending in the

15

Total = $30,828 million

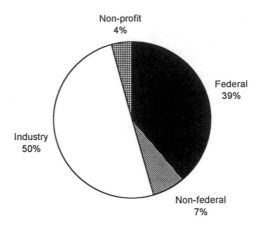

FIGURE 2-1 Health R&D funding by source, 1993. SOURCE: U.S. Department of Health and Human Services, 1993.

health-related components of federal agencies,[1] principally the National Institutes of Health (NIH) in the Department of Health and Human Services (DHHS), represented nearly $12 billion, or 39 percent of all spending (see Figure 2-1). Spending by state and local governments contributed about $2 billion, or slightly less than 7 percent of national spending on health R&D.

The difference, $17 billion or 54 percent, is financed by health R&D spending in the private sector—primarily industry, but also private nonprofit organizations such as the Howard Hughes Medical Institute and other foundations. Industry was the largest single sponsor of biomedical R&D in 1993, financing in excess of 50 percent of all biomedical R&D (although, as we will see, the nature of this R&D is different in several respects from research funded by federal spending). Total expenditures by private, nonprofit institutions (including universities) for health R&D were $1.2 billion, or 4 percent of all spending (see Figure 2-1). In addition to this explicit investment of institutional funds, universities also support biomedical R&D through cross-subsidization from patient-care dollars. It has recently been estimated that the amount of such subsidies is around $850 million.

---

[1]Health R&D is defined as "biomedical, health services, and other health-related R&D projects, resources, and general support, but not training or construction." See U.S. Department of Health and Human Services, 1993.

Federal Spending for Biomedical Research and Development

The phenomenon of large-scale public support for biomedical research in the United States is relatively recent. In 1940, for example, the largest funders of biomedical research performed in the United States were corporations and non-profit organizations, spending $25 million and $17 million, respectively (not adjusted for the effects of inflation). Spending by federal agencies for biomedical research was largely in their own laboratories and equaled only $3 million, or less than 7 percent of all spending (Ginzberg and Dutka, 1989).

From a policy perspective, the expansion of public sector spending for biomedical research can be traced to the dramatic advances achieved by academic research during the 1930s and 1940s, such as the development of radar and the jet engine but also important advances in medicine, including the discovery by Fleming and then development by Flory and Heatley of penicillin to treat infectious disease (see Ginzberg and Dutka, 1989; Rosenberg and Nelson, 1993). Increasingly, basic research was seen as important to social goals, including improved health, and consequently deserving of public sector support. This view was successfully articulated by Vannevar Bush in an influential report, *Science— the Endless Frontier*, that proposed large-scale public sector funding for basic research, including significant support for biomedical R&D (Bush, 1945). As a consequence of this view, public sector spending for biomedical research, as well as for academic research in all areas, increased enormously as illustrated in Figure 2-2. From 1950 to 1965, appropriations to NIH to expand the funding of

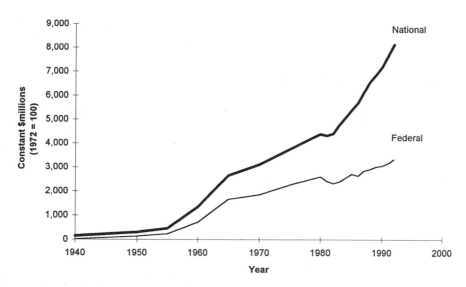

FIGURE 2-2 National and federal funds for health R&D, 1940–1992. SOURCE: Ginzberg and Dutka, 1989; U.S. DHHS, 1993.

biomedical research accelerated in real terms at 18 percent annually, eclipsing spending by corporations and nonprofit organizations (Ginzberg and Dutka, 1989). By 1965, federal spending had become the source of nearly two out of every three dollars spent on biomedical research, largely through programs of NIH.

More recently, federal funding of biomedical research has continued to follow a trend of real, sometimes substantial, increases over inflation. From 1983 to 1993, federal spending for biomedical research increased from $5.4 billion to $12.0 billion in current dollars, or 36 percent adjusting for the effects of inflation[2] (U.S. DHHS, 1993). Federal spending for *basic* research in the life sciences increased by more than $3.3 billion[3] (National Science Board, 1993). Indeed, the percentage increase in funding for the life sciences over this period was exceeded only by spending for research in mathematics and computer science, although in absolute terms the increase in these areas is comparatively small ($0.35 billion) (Laubach, 1994; National Science Board, 1993).

Despite these increases in federal spending, national spending for biomedical research has increased even faster. From 1983 to 1993, national spending from *all* sources increased $20 billion, or more than 75 percent (adjusted for the effects of inflation; U.S. DHHS, 1993). During this time period, the significance of federal funding has changed. Figure 2-3 illustrates that relative levels of federal spending are decreasing, from 50 percent of all funding in 1983 to 39 percent in 1993 (even though federal spending for biomedical research, in absolute terms, has increased).

For 1994, $11.4 billion of the $71.6 billion that the federal government was projected to spend on general scientific R&D was to support biomedical research and development (up 6.5 percent from FY 1993;[4] American Association for the Advancement of Science, 1993a). NIH appropriations are about 90 percent of this spending[5] (see Table 2-1). In addition to NIH, agencies that sponsor academic biomedical research include the National Science Foundation, the Centers for Disease Control and Prevention, the Department of Veterans Affairs, the Department of Defense, and the Department of Energy. Most of this spending by federal agencies is directed to extramural programs as opposed to research in

---

[2]Constant dollars based on the Biomedical R&D Price Index (U.S. DHHS, 1993).

[3]Federal obligations for basic research in (1) biological sciences (excluding environmental) and (2) medical sciences. See Appendix table 4-15, in National Science Board, 1993.

[4]These figures use health spending for DHHS, Department of Veterans Affairs, and the Department of Education; they are not comparable to NIH data, which include the health-related components of all agencies' R&D, irrespective of their formal budget classifications.

[5]Three institutes of the Alcohol, Drug Abuse, and Mental Health Administration (ADAMHA)—the National Institute of Mental Health, the National Institute on Drug Abuse, and the National Institute on Alcohol Abuse and Alcoholism—were merged into NIH in 1993 as independent institutes. NIH figures for 1994 are adjusted to include the funding for these institutes. See AAAS, 1993b.

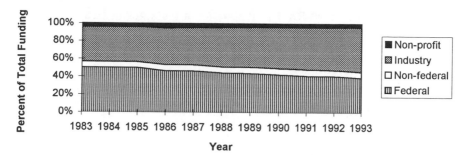

FIGURE 2-3 Trends in sources of funding for biomedical R&D as a percent of total R&D funds, 1983–1993. SOURCE: U.S. Department of Health and Human Services, 1993.

federal laboratories.   Universities and academic medical centers are the largest recipients of these extramural funds, receiving nearly 75 percent of all extramural spending (see Figure 2-4; U.S. DHHS, 1993).

Federal Spending for Medical Device Research and Development

Medical devices (a primary focus of this volume) are different from pharmaceuticals and biotechnology in that they constitute a relatively small item within the federal medical research budget. This is because they draw heavily on advances in physics and engineering (see Gelijns and Rosenberg, chapter 1 of this volume).   For this reason, the focus on basic advances in disease- and organ-specific research in university research funded by NIH has largely excluded medical device development (Foote, 1992).   A recent study estimates that federal spending for biomedical R&D in these areas accounted for only about $422 million in 1992, a decrease of $27 million from 1991 spending (see Table 2-2). Of this, three-quarters was funded by NIH spending (less than 5 percent of NIH appropriations).

There are exceptions to this—appropriations by Congress to NIH are occasionally targeted to specific technologies or systems that require medical device development. Examples include the Artificial Heart Program and the Artificial Kidney Program (Foote, 1992). More recently, the Human Genome Project has specifically solicited interdisciplinary proposals both for developing advanced sequencing and mapping technology and for computational methods to organize and analyze the resulting data (IOM, 1990).   In addition to these programs, the National Science Foundation also funds investigator-initiated research in a number of areas that are relevant to innovation in medical devices, including several programs in science and biological engineering (IOM, 1990).   As a group, though, these programs represent a relatively small percentage of the university biomedical research enterprise.

TABLE 2-1   Estimated R&D in the National Institutes of Health (in million dollars)

Topic	FY 1993 (est.)	FY 1994 (approved)	Percent Increase
Cancer	1,978.3	2,082.3	5.26
Heart, Lung, and Blood	1,214.7	1,277.9	5.20
Dental Research	161.1	169.5	5.21
Diabetes, Digestive, and Kidney Diseases	680.7	716.1	5.20
Neurological Disorders and Stroke	599.5	630.7	5.20
Allergy and Infectious Disease	988.4	1,065.6	7.81
General Medical Sciences	832.2	875.5	5.20
Child Health and Human Development	527.8	555.2	5.19
Eye	275.9	290.3	5.22
Environmental Health Services	251.2	264.2	5.18
Aging	399.5	420.3	5.21
Arthritis and Musculoskeletal and Skin Diseases	212.2	223.3	5.23
Deafness and Communications Disorders	154.8	162.8	5.17
Research Resources	312.7	331.9	6.14
Nursing Research	48.5	51	5.15
Alcoholism and Alcohol Abuse	176.4	185.6	5.22
Drug Abuse	404.2	425.2	5.20
Mental Health	583.1	613.4	5.20
Human Genome	106.1	128.7	21.30
Fogarty International Center	19.7	21.7	10.15
National Library of Medicine	103.6	120	15.83
Office of Director	190.3	233.6	22.75
Buildings and Facilities	108.7	111	2.12
TOTAL, NIH Budget	10,329.6	10,955.8	6.06
Estimated Research Training	(349.0)	(373.4)	6.99
Other non-R&D	(90.6)	(107.6)	18.76
TOTAL, NIH R&D	9,890.0	10,474.8	5.91

NOTE: Includes AAAS estimates of (a) conduct of R&D, and (b) R&D facilities. FY, fiscal year.

SOURCE: American Association for the Advancement of Science (AAAS), 1993a.

A Change in the Emphasis of Federal Spending

In recent years, concern in Congress over the federal deficit and efforts to control the increase in federal spending have created increased competition for appropriations and focused attention explicitly on the results of public spending for biomedical research; NIH's National Cancer Institute, for example, was recently chastised for failing after 20 years of large-scale public spending to dem-

Total = $11,727 million

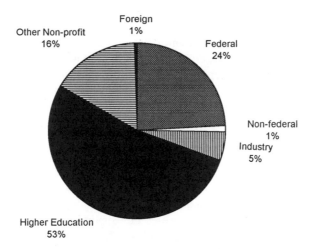

FIGURE 2-4 Distribution of federal health R&D funding by performer, 1992. SOURCE: U.S. Department of Health and Human Services, 1993.

TABLE 2-2   Estimated Federal Spending for Medical Device-related R&D (in million dollars)

Agency	FY 1991	FY 1992	Percent Change
National Institutes of Health	378.9	354.4	−6
National Science Foundation	18.0	18.0	0
Department of Defense	22.8	15.0	−34
Department of Veterans Affairs	9.3	10.5	13
Food and Drug Administration	9.4	10.2	9
Department of Energy	2.7	5.8	115
National Aeronautics and Space Administration	4.9	4.9	0
Department of Education	2.3	2.3	0
National Institutes of Standards and Technology	0.5	0.5	0
TOTAL	448.8	421.6	−6

SOURCE: Littell, 1994.

onstrate more significant results in the prevention and treatment of cancer (AAAS, 1992).

This trend not only exists within biomedicine, but also in other sectors of the economy (AAAS, 1993a). It reflects the view that in many areas of high technology the globalization of research and the pressure of international competition have introduced a critical time dimension into the stream of product development (NAS, 1992; Office of Science and Technology Policy, 1994). Whereas the United States has enjoyed a competitive advantage in many high technology fields, there is a perception that other countries may have developed more effective means for the direct translation of new knowledge into commercial products. As indicated by a number of forums, reports, and congressional hearings, the consequence of this view is that federal funding for research will become increasingly tied to societal goals. The same emphasis has been echoed by the Carnegie Commission on Science, Technology, and Government (1992).

Several programmatic consequences of this thinking can be identified in the FY 1994 budget. First, new federal research support appears to be concentrated in particular areas of science and technology seen as critical to national goals. These initiatives and their proposed funding levels in the FY 1994 budget are biotechnology research ($4.3 billion, largely through NIH), advanced materials and processing ($2.1 billion), global environmental change research ($1.5 billion), advanced manufacturing technology ($1.4 billion), high-performance computing and communications ($1.0 billion), and science, mathematics, and engineering technology education ($2.3 billion) (National Science Board, 1993).

Second, within NIH this increased focus on the economic and social benefits of publicly-funded biomedical research is expressed in a growing number of focused initiatives required by Congress or the administration (National Science Commission, 1992; Anderson, 1993). For example, the administration explicitly targeted several research initiatives for increased funding in its proposed budget to Congress for fiscal year 1994 (AAAS, 1993b). These initiatives and the proposed funding levels include AIDS research ($1.3 billion), women's health ($61 million, as part of a 15-year project estimated to cost over $650 million), breast cancer research ($216 million), and minority health ($56 million).

Direct Federal Support for Industry

Of the 30 percent of extramural funds not received by universities and medical schools, one-third (11 percent of all extramural funds) was used to fund biomedical R&D in industry in 1992 (see Figure 2-4). These extramural funds represented 6 percent of biomedical R&D performed by industry (U.S. DHHS, 1993).

These funds do not only flow through NIH. The National Institute of Standards and Technology (NIST), for example, is the focus of new spending for applied research and development in several areas, including biomedical R&D.

The NIST component with the largest increase in funding in FY 1994 was the Advanced Technology Program (ATP), which partially funds research and development in individual companies and joint ventures to develop promising, high-risk technologies, where the risks are perceived as too high to pursue without the incentive of federal spending. As examples, projects recently funded by ATP include development of synthetic polymers as bio-absorbable materials for use in orthopedics; development of implantable "microreactors," containing living cells that are isolated from the body's immune system, to treat diseases requiring bioagents produced by the cells; and the use of multi-photon detector technology to develop radioisotope detection and measurement systems for use in diagnostics (AAAMI, 1994b; AAAS, 1993b). ATP's budget in FY 1994 was $199.5 million (AAAS, 1993a; Robinson, 1994).

At the same time, spending for defense programs is increasingly expected to promote dual-use technology development. In this context, the FY 1994 budget designated the Advanced Research Projects Agency as the lead agency for the Technology Reinvestment Project (TRP) in dual-use technologies, intended to help smaller defense contractors develop technologies for defense that also have commercial applications. Total funding for the TRP initiative is $472 million (AAAS, 1993b; Robinson, 1994). The initiative is divided into 11 technology areas, one of which is health care technology. Medical projects funded under TRP include a prototype ceramic honeycomb system that will separate oxygen from air and deliver the oxygen under pressure without pumps or moving parts; and a consortium in commercializing computer-vision technology originally developed for the National Aeronautics and Space Administration (NASA; AAAMI, 1994e).

In addition to the ATP and TRP initiatives, federal funding also explicitly targets applied research in smaller, technology-intensive companies through the Small Business Innovation Research (SBIR) program started in 1983. Under this program, when a federal agency's extramural research spending exceeds $100 million the agency is required to set aside a fixed percentage of this spending for SBIR projects. SBIR divides research support into three phases. Phase 1 awards are up to $100,000 and are used to evaluate the scientific and technical usefulness of an idea. In Phase 2, projects from Phase 1 with demonstrated potential are funded up to $750,000 to further develop the proposed idea for one or two years. Phase 3 aims for commercialization by private sector investment; no SBIR funds may be used for this purpose. In 1994, NIH set aside 1.5 percent ($125 million) for SBIR awards in the life sciences. For FY 1995, this increases to 2 percent (about $165-170 million), and increases for FY 1997 to 2.5 percent (about $230 million) (AAAMI, 1994c; Robinson, 1994).

The newest program for FY 1994 is the Small Business Technology Transfer (SBTT) program, also intended explicitly to help small business. SBTT is distinct from SBIR in that SBTT also aims to encourage cooperative R&D and technology transfer between small businesses and research institutions. Consequently, small businesses are required to team with research institutions to receive SBTT funding (no such requirement exists for SBIR). SBTT began a three year pilot program in FY 1994. Funding levels for SBTT were also initially below the levels for SBIR. In 1994, this amounted to $4.1 million for NIH, or approximately 40 awards in FY 1994 (AAAMI, 1994c).

Tax Credits on Incremental Research and Development

As well as direct federal funding to support biomedical research, substantial indirect support for research is provided to industry in the form of tax credits on incremental R&D expenses. According to estimates by the U.S. Treasury Department, this indirect means of federal support for basic R&D has accounted for more than $20 billion from 1981 to 1992 (National Science Board, 1993). No data are available specifically for biomedical R&D. Unfortunately, a tax credit requires positive earnings, not usually enjoyed by the smaller, innovative companies in biotechnology or medical devices.

Industry Spending for Biomedical Research and Development

The largest source of financing for biomedical R&D is spending from private sources. As illustrated in Figure 2-1 above, industry is the main supporter of biomedical R&D in the United States. Industry spending exceeded $15 billion in 1993, or 50 percent of all health R&D, and substantially exceeded all sources of federal financing, including NIH. Industry spending was also the most rapidly increasing source of financing in 1993 (U.S. DHHS, 1993).

Industry performed by far the majority (78 percent) of the $15 billion in biomedical R&D that it funded in 1993 (see Figure 2-5), as well as 40 percent of all spending on health R&D overall (U.S. DHHS, 1993). For-profit sponsorship of research at universities and academic medical centers remains a relatively small proportion of the total investment by industry in R&D. According to the American Association for the Advancement of Science, about 11 percent of funds received by universities in 1991, or $1.35 billion, come from industry; only 5 percent of industrial R&D is allocated for basic or fundamental research (AAAS, 1993b).

Research and Development Investments by
Pharmaceutical and Biotechnology Companies

The pharmaceutical sector is the largest industrial funder of biomedical R&D. According to the Pharmaceutical Manufacturers Association (PMA; 1993b), there were 136 pharmaceutical companies operating in the United States in 1993. The member companies of the PMA, representing over 90 percent of U.S. pharmaceutical sales, spent $12.6 billion on biomedical R&D in 1993

Total = $13,870 million

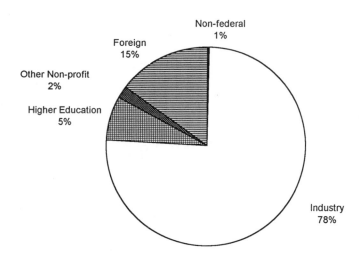

FIGURE 2-5 Distribution of industry health R&D funding by performer, 1992. SOURCE: U.S. DHHS, 1993.

(PMA, 1993b). R&D spending for PMA members has also accelerated faster than federal spending for biomedical R&D, increasing on average 14 percent per year starting in 1970 (see Figure 2-6). This spending for R&D represents about 17 percent of total pharmaceutical sales, or more than double the percentage of R&D spending in other technology-intensive sectors of the U.S. economy (U.S. Department of Commerce, 1994).

Research performed in company laboratories represents over 75 percent of this spending on R&D—about 25 percent is contracted to outside organizations, including universities and academic medical centers (PMA, 1993b). Most R&D spending is in four areas—cardiovasculars, drugs related to the central nervous system, anti-infectives, and neoplasms (PMA, 1993b). Clinical evaluation phases I through IV comprise about 30 percent of R&D spending, and probably represent the largest component of industry funding to universities and academic medical centers (PMA, 1993b).

The nature of this research is changing. According to a recent study of the pharmaceutical industry by the Boston Consulting Group (BCG), more than two-thirds of all drugs in development are now aimed at chronic diseases (BCG, 1993). The effects of this changing focus are reflected in the greater complexity and difficulty of pharmaceutical R&D—especially the lack of clear clinical end-points to demonstrate efficacy and longer and larger clinical trials (BCG, 1993). Figures 2-7 and 2-8 show the rate at which clinical trials have increased in duration and size. The rapidly changing health care environment places a premium on

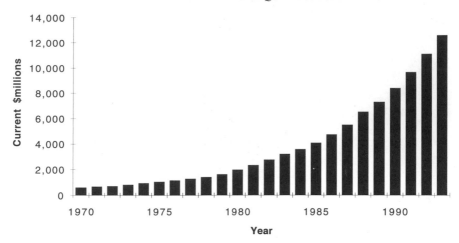

FIGURE 2-6 Total R&D spending, Pharmaceutical Manufacturers Association member companies, 1990–1993. SOURCE: PMA, 1993b.

truly novel drugs. Within this context, the distinction between pharmaceutical companies and biotechnology companies is blurring as pharmaceutical companies are increasingly using biotechnology techniques to develop new drugs. According to the BCG study, 33 percent of research projects in major pharmaceutical companies in 1993 were based on biotechnology, compared with only 2 percent in 1980. In some larger pharmaceutical companies, up to 70 percent of the research projects were based on molecular biology (BCG, 1993).

According to a recent "DataWatch" article in *Health Affairs*, the biotechnology sector included 1,272 biotechnology companies in 1993, of which 235 are public (Read and Lee, 1994). More than 100 of these companies were started in the last two years. Compared to the larger pharmaceutical sector, biotechnology is relatively small—according to a survey by Ernst and Young (1994), revenues for biotechnology companies were about $7 billion in 1992, compared to revenues of $114 billion for pharmaceutical companies. The biotechnology sector is nonetheless a very large funder of biomedical research. According to the same survey, biotechnology companies spent nearly $5.7 billion on R&D in 1992 (or about half the R&D expenditures for pharmaceuticals), or nearly 80 percent of sales (Read and Lee, 1994). As is obvious from these levels of R&D spending, the overwhelming majority of biotechnology companies are research organizations with essentially no revenues. Moreover, with very few exceptions, development efforts in the majority of these biotechnology companies are several years from approval. Table 2-3 shows the number of drugs currently in development that use biotechnology techniques, including drugs developed by larger pharmaceutical companies. Currently, there are only 19 biotechnology drugs approved for use in the United States (see Table 2-4).

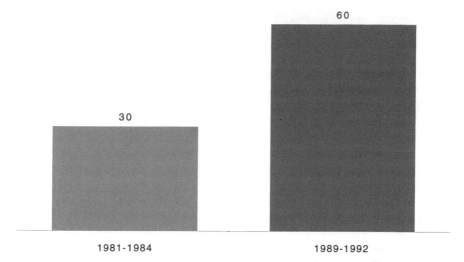

FIGURE 2-7 Average number of clinical trials per New Drug Application to the Food and Drug Administration. SOURCE: Boston Consulting Group, 1993.

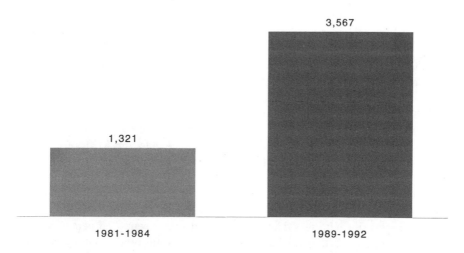

FIGURE 2-8 Average number of patients per clinical trial. SOURCE: Boston Consulting Group, 1993.

TABLE 2-3   Biotechnology Drugs Currently in Development

	1989	1990	1991	1993
Approved medicines	9	11	14	19
Medicines or vaccines in development				
Phase I	26	38	48	41
Phase I/II	12	13	16	22
Phase II	23	32	46	53
Phase II/III	8	6	7	6
Phase III	11	15	18	33
Phase not specified	5	3	2	4
Application at FDA for review	10	19	21	11
TOTAL medicines or vaccines in development	95	126	158	170

NOTE: Total medicines or vaccines in development reflects medicines in development for more than one indication.

SOURCE: PMA, *Biotechnology Medicines in Development*, 1993.

Research and Development Investments by the Medical Devices Industry

In contrast to pharmaceuticals and biotechnology, medical devices encompass a more diverse group of products, ranging from disposable needles to sophisticated and expensive modalities such as magnetic resonance imaging (MRI). At present, the Food and Drug Administration (FDA) identifies about 1,700 different types of medical devices, which are developed and manufactured by as many as 11,000 device companies (including foreign companies; Gelijns et al., forthcoming). According to the U.S. Department of Commerce, surgical and medical instruments, surgical appliances and supplies, electromedical equipment, and X-ray equipment were projected to be among the fastest growing sectors of U.S. industry in 1993 (U.S. Department of Commerce, 1993).

In 1993, the medical device industry invested less than 7 percent of sales in R&D, compared to 17 percent in pharmaceuticals (*Business Week*, 1994). Large variations in R&D spending exist among device categories, however, reflecting the complexity of the type of product involved—developing MRI, of course, is considerably more complicated than developing a new set of surgical instruments. R&D spending also varies depending on company size, mirroring the division of labor between large pharmaceutical companies and biotechnology companies. According to an analysis by the Health Care Technology Institute, device companies with less than $5 million in sales spent 77.5 percent of their sales in 1991 on R&D, or almost the identical figure for biotechnology (although the absolute level of spending is almost certainly less). This spending for R&D compares to 17.2 percent for companies with between $5 and $20 million in

TABLE 2-4 Biotechnology Medicines or Vaccines Approved by the Food and Drug Administration, 1993

Product	Indications	Company	Year Approved
Beta interferon	Multiple sclerosis	Chiron	1993
DNAse	Cystic fibrosis	Genentech	1993
Factor VIII	Hemophilia	Genentech, Genetics Institute	1993
IL-2	Renal cell cancer	Chiron	1992
Indium-111-labeled antibody	Cancer imaging	Cytogen	1992
Aglucerase	Gaucher's disease	Genzyme	1991
G-CSF	Adjunct to chemotherapy	Amgen	1991
GM-CSF	Bone marrow transplant	Immunex	1991
Hyaluronic acid	Ophthalmic surgery	Genzyme	1991
CMV immune globulin	Prevention of rejection in organ transplants	MedImmune	1990
Gamma interferon	Chronic granulomatous disease	Genentech	1990
PEG-adenosine deaminase	Immune deficiency	Enzon	1990
t-PA	Myocardial infarction, pulmonary embolism	Genentech	1990
Erythropoietin	Anemia associated with renal failure, AIDS, cancer	Amgen	1989
Hepatitis B antigens	Diagnosis	Biogen	1987
Alpha interferon	Cancer, genital warts, hepatitis	Biogen, Genentech	1986
Hepatitis B vaccine	Prevention	Biogen, Chiron	1986
Human growth hormone	Deficiency	Genentech	1985
Human insulin	Type I diabetes	Genentech	1982

SOURCE: "Datawatch: Biotechnology and Innovation Progress Reports," in *Health Affairs*, Summer, 1994.

sales, and 4.5 percent for companies with greater than $100 million in sales (Health Care Technology Institute, 1993).

FUNDING RELATIONSHIPS BETWEEN INDUSTRY AND UNIVERSITIES

Over the past decade, the number and variety of industry-university relationships has increased dramatically. The two most common forms of collaboration between industry and academia for biomedical R&D are project-specific research support, and consulting arrangements (Blumenthal, 1994). Other frequent types of collaboration—including large-scale investments in academic research centers by industry—have received much more attention, perhaps because of their novelty in the life sciences (Atkinson, 1994). A list compiled by Webster and Etzkowitz of large-scale collaborations between pharmaceutical companies and academia through 1990 is reproduced in Table 2-5.

Despite the dramatic increase in attention to and interest in relationships between universities and industry, there is no centralized source of data to track consulting arrangements or the amount of project-specific biomedical R&D that industry funds in universities (Committee on Small Business, March 11, 1993). Estimates do exist for the subset of university research involving biotechnology techniques, however. Estimates by Blumenthal indicate that industry funding of individual research projects in academia totaled between $85 million and $135 million in 1984, or between 8 and 24 percent of all funds available for biotechnology research in academia (Blumenthal, 1992). These estimates also indicate that spending per project was less than the average size of NIH grants, and that these projects were typically of a shorter duration, suggesting that industry-sponsored research may be more focused and applied in nature than research funded by federal spending (Blumenthal et al., 1986).

Beyond industry funding of individual projects, faculty at major research-intensive universities performing research in biotechnology also receive support through consulting arrangements with industry. According to Blumenthal, 47 percent of biotechnology faculty had consulted for industry at some point over a three-year period ending in 1984 (Blumenthal, 1992). In a separate survey of nearly 700 graduate students and fellows in life sciences departments at six leading universities, 19 percent received some research or educational support from industry (Blumenthal, 1992).

FEDERAL EFFORTS TO ENCOURAGE TECHNOLOGY TRANSFER

Over the past decade, federal legislation has been introduced to encourage collaborations between universities and industry and to improve and extend these interactions. This legislation recognizes that industry must have reasonable expectations of being able to recover its development costs, which may be consid-

TABLE 2-5 Selected Large-scale Relationships Between Universities/Academic Health Centers and Industry in Biomedical Research (in million dollars)

University/Academic Health Center	Industry Partner	Funds (million$)	Duration	Started	Focus
Harvard University Medical School	Takeda	1.0 per annum	Open-ended	1986	Angiogenesis factors
Washington University	Monsanto	100.0	12	1982	Biomedical research
Massachusetts General Hospital	Shiseido	85.0	1	1989	Dermatology
Massachusetts General Hospital	Hoechst	70.0	12	1981	Molecular biology
Georgetown University	Fidia	62.0	Open-ended	1985	Neurosciences
Massachusetts General Hospital	Bristol-Myers Squibb	37.0	5	1990	Cardiovascular
Harvard University Medical School	Monsanto	23.5	12	1974	Cancer angiogenesis
University of California at San Diego	Ciba Geigy	20.0	6	1990	Rheumatoid and osteoarthritis
Harvard University Medical School	Hoffman-LaRoche	10.0	5	1990	Medicinal chemistry
Harvard University Medical School	DuPont	6.0	5	1981	Genetics
Washington University	Mallink	3.8	5	1981	Hybridomas
Yale University	Bristol-Myers	3.0	5	1982	Anticancer drugs
Columbia University	Bristol-Myers	2.3	6	1983	Gene structure
Johns Hopkins University	SmithKline Beckman	2.2	5	1988	Respiratory disease
Yale University	Celanese	1.1	5	1981	Enzymes
Johns Hopkins University	Johnson & Johnson	1.0	Open-ended	1982	Biology
Rochester University	Kodak (Sterling)	0.5	Open-ended	1983	DNA

SOURCE: Statement of J. L. Wagner and M. E. Gluck, OTA, to the U.S. Congress Subcommittee on Business Opportunities, Regulation, and Energy of the House Committee on Small Business. Adapted from A. J. Webster and H. Etzkowitz, *Academic-Industry Relations, The Second Academic Revolution: A Framework Paper for the Proposed Workshop on Academic-Industry Relations* (London, England, Science Policy Support Group, 1991).

erable, or it will not participate. Patents and licenses on intellectual property developed at universities are, consequently, important for the transfer of technologies, and especially biotechnology, to clinical practice (Committee on Small Business, 1993b; IOM, 1989).

The Stevenson-Wydler and the Bayh-Dole Acts

The first element of this legislative effort is the 1980 Stevenson-Wydler Technology Transfer Act. Broadly, Stevenson-Wydler established an infrastructure for technology transfer from federal laboratories into the universities and industry. To facilitate technology transfer the act requires that each agency with federal laboratories allocate 0.5 percent of the agency research and development budget for this purpose. Federal laboratories having an annual budget exceeding $20 million are also required to provide at least one full-time professional position dedicated to this function (Chen, 1993; IOM, 1989). Despite the failure of Congress to appropriate funds for Stevenson-Wydler, other congressional and executive actions followed which reinforced the policy that federal agencies should actively pursue collaborative relationships with private industry.

The second example of such legislation is the 1980 Bayh-Dole Patent and Trademark Laws Amendment. Essentially, Bayh-Dole enables intellectual property rights to discoveries made using federal funds to be assigned to the university or research institution. It also allows the institution to seek patents and, in turn, to license and collect royalties on these patents, as long as these funds are used for scientific research and are shared with the principal investigator (Chen, 1993).

The apparent effect of Stevenson-Wydler and Bayh-Dole on academic biomedical research is impressive, at least in terms of patents. According to a study performed by the General Accounting Office (GAO), the top 35 research universities (all among the 25 leading recipients of NIH and NSF support during 1989-1990) accounted for 2,043 patent applications and 1,063 patents; of these, 731 were licensed, representing more than $113 million in income from licenses. The majority of these patents and licenses were in the health sciences (Blumenthal, 1992). Indeed, in biotechnology, universities were more efficient in generating patents than private industry—biotechnology companies in the 1980s were realizing more than four times as many patent applications per dollar invested from university research than from their own labs (Blumenthal, 1992).

Federal Technology Transfer Act

The 1986 Federal Technology Transfer Act extended the ideas in Bayh-Dole about university-industry relationships to interactions between federal laboratories and industry. The law authorizes the directors of federal labs to negotiate licensing agreements for inventions made in federal labs, and for the licensing fees and royalties to be shared with the federal employee/inventor, the remainder to be retained by the laboratory for technology transfer (Chen, 1993; IOM, 1989). Incentives are also offered for companies and federal laboratories to enter into cooperative research and development agreements (Chen, 1993).

It should be stressed that these federal efforts in biomedical research are not restricted to NIH. In addition to NIH, several other agencies sponsor intramural research in technologies that may be relevant to the development, in particular, of medical devices. Several medical technologies developed under contract for NASA, for example, have been successfully transferred to clinical use, including a compliant knee joint for prosthetic and robotic devices that permits rotational movement in three different planes, and a walker for dynamically supporting persons with limited use of their extremities (AAAMI, 1994d).

To encourage the transfer of these technologies and expertise from the federal laboratories (in all areas, not only biomedical research), the National Technology Transfer Center (NTTC) was started in 1993 using a five-year grant from NASA. The intent of NTTC is to transfer technologies from the national laboratories, including NASA, into the commercial sector. NTTC is currently linked to more than 700 federal laboratories at 17 federal agencies, and serves as an electronic "gateway" to federal research resources, via searches of available technologies (AAAMI, 1994a).

Consequences for University-Industry Relationships

The trends in funding for biomedical R&D identified in this chapter have had remarkable consequences for research universities. First, the scale of the academic research enterprise has increased enormously, in all disciplines. As the universities have expanded their research programs to absorb the increased federal spending for research, the size and complexity of the research enterprise have created an economic imperative for the larger research universities. For example, Columbia University has seen a doubling of budget size every 10 years, and expenses increasing at 10 percent compounded annually for the past forty-five years (Cole, 1993). In academic biomedical research, spending by the leading research universities and medical schools has also increased nearly 200 times in response to increases in NIH support for basic and clinical research, from $50 million in 1950 to $9.7 billion in 1993 (nearly 30 times in constant dollars; Ginzberg and Dutka, 1989; U.S. DHHS, 1993).

Federal financing of academic biomedical research is critical for the long-term development of the research base and for immediate program funding. Nonetheless, the emphasis of appropriations for biomedical R&D has shifted, increasing the level of spending required to support the research enterprise but no longer permitting major expansion (AAAS, 1993b). Consequently, universities are seeking new sources of capital to maintain and expand (selectively) the base of academic research.

For major research universities, one of these sources is licensing fees realized under the Stevenson-Wydler and Bayh-Dole acts, especially in the emerging field of biotechnology. The patent on DNA recombinant techniques by Boyer and Cohen is a particularly lucrative example: income from the Cohen-Boyer patents for 1991–1992 represented $14.6 million, or 58 percent of total income from all patents held by Stanford University (total income for 1991–1992 was $25.5 million). The GAO survey of the top 35 universities cited earlier does raise questions as to whether this is a useful source of financing for more than a few universities, however. The universities surveyed reported an average income from licenses of $1.6 million; nine universities reported income in excess of $1.0 million and only six reported income in excess of $2.0 million (Blumenthal, 1992). The relatively few commercially profitable inventions emerging from those institutions and the substantial minimum efficient scale of operation, ". . . [imply] there is a reasonably high probability that many universities that 'invest' in expanded technology licensing operations in order to produce substantial new sources of income [will fail]" (Feller, 1990, p. 340).

In response to increasing biomedical research opportunities, many larger research universities have also directly or indirectly established ventures to commercialize their academic research. In a recent issue of *Health Affairs*, Atkinson discussed the university-based venture capital funds that were established at Harvard, Johns Hopkins, and Columbia Universities (Atkinson, 1994). Critics of these arrangements have questioned whether true organizational separation is possible—Harvard University, for example, had rejected a 1980 proposal to invest in a start-up biotechnology firm intended to develop research by a Harvard faculty member because it was considered incompatible with the university's central mission of learning. "The preservation of academic values is a matter of paramount importance to the University," wrote Derek Bok, then president of Harvard University, "and owning shares in a company would create a number of potential conflicts of interest with these values" (Hunnewell, 1994). In 1988, however, the university reversed itself by establishing Medical Science Partners, an enterprise designed to commercialize biomedical research findings. More recently, Harvard has proposed to establish an academic research center, the Harvard Institutes of Medicine, that will also include biotechnology companies (Hunnewell, 1994). In both instances, the university has faced little of the faculty criticism or media attention that accompanied the 1980 proposal. To date, however, no evidence is available on whether these university-based venture capital funds are in fact an effective means of commercializing research findings.

CONCLUDING OBSERVATIONS

Increased investments in R&D have contributed to the development of new knowledge; the strengthening of the pharmaceutical and device industries; the growth of universities, academic health centers, and medical specialties; and the emergence of the biotechnology industry. The recent science policy statement, *Science in the National Interest*, reaffirms the federal investment in science, ". . . both to sustain America's preeminence in science and to facilitate the role of science in the broader national interest" (OSTP, 1994). Technological innovations both to improve and preserve health and to assure economic prosperity are strong and continuing rationales for investments in R&D.

In recent years, the rapid proliferation of collaborations in biological research involving partnerships between universities, industry, and government have greatly extended the frequency, scope, and visibility of such activities. The desire to draw commercial potential out of government-supported science has led to legislative and executive initiatives to promote more frequent and more directed technology transfer collaborations between the sectors. In many instances, as mentioned, it is still too soon to know how effective the different initiatives will be in fostering technology transfer. Continued monitoring and evaluation to assess what works should guide future policy development.

The amounts of dollars contributed for funding of science by the different sectors have changed over the past decade. While at one time government was the major investor in science, today industry supports over 50 percent of health R&D. It seems likely that the federal government will continue to support biomedical R&D handsomely, though perhaps not the continued expansion of the American university system. Consequently, if there is to be future growth of academic research it will depend increasingly on industrial support. Future policies will need to create an environment favorable to such private sector support. As we have noted, federal policies such as those governing intellectual property rights or tax credits for investments in R&D affect the level of support for R&D and the relationships of the different sectors. Furthermore, as U.S. scientists in academia seek more money from industrial sources, such collaborations will raise questions about potential conflicts of interest and about the roles of universities in education and in economic prosperity. Efforts to regulate collaboration between the sectors should seek to eliminate these ambiguities without unnecessarily burdening university-industry agreements.

REFERENCES

American Association for the Advancement of Medical Instrumentation (AAAMI). 1994a. National center facilitates technology transfer. In: *Medical Device Research Report* 1(1):11. Arlington, Va.: AAAMI.

AAAMI. 1994b. NIST Advanced Technology Program seeks proposals. In: *Medical Device Research Report* 1(2):6. Arlington, Va.: AAAMI.

AAAMI. 1994c. SBIR, STTR funding opportunities at NIH. In: *Medical Device Research Report* 1(1):3–5. Arlington, Va.: AAAMI.

AAAMI. 1994d. Technologies available. In: *Medical Device Research Report* 1(2):13. Arlington, Va.: AAAMI.

AAAMI. 1994e. Technology Reinvestment Project aims to develop 'dual-use' technolo-

36 ENRIQUETA C. BOND AND SIMON GLYNN

gies. In: *Medical Device Research Report* 1(2):2. Arlington, Va.: AAAMI.

American Association for the Advancement of Science (AAAS). 1992. *Research and Development FY 1992.* Publication no. 91-17S. Washington, D.C.: AAAS.

AAAS. 1993a. *Congressional Action on Research and Development in the FY 1994 Budget.* Publication No. 93-35S. Washington, D.C.: AAAS.

AAAS. 1993b. *Research and Development FY 1994.* Publication No. 93-10S. Washington, D.C.: AAAS.

Anderson, C. 1993. Strategic research wins the day. *Science* 259:21.

Atkinson, S. H. 1994. University-affiliated venture capital funds. *Health Affairs* (Summer):159–175.

Blumenthal, D. 1992. Academic-industry relationships in the life sciences. *Journal of the American Medical Association* 268:3344–3349.

Blumenthal, D. 1994. Growing pains for new academic/industry relationships. *Health Affairs* (Summer):176–193.

Blumenthal, D., Gluck, M., Louis, K., et al. 1986. University-industry research relationships in biotechnology: Implications for the university. *Science* 232:1361–1366.

Boston Consulting Group (BCG). 1993. *The Changing Environment for U.S. Pharmaceuticals: The Role of Pharmaceutical Companies in a Systems Approach to Health Care.* Boston, Mass.: BCG.

Bush, V. 1945. *Science—The Endless Frontier. A Report to the President on a Program for Postwar Scientific Research.* Washington, D.C.: Office of Scientific Research and Development.

Business Week. 1994. R&D Scoreboard. June 27, pp. 78–103.

Carnegie Commission on Science, Technology, and Government. 1992. *Enabling the Future: Linking Science and Technology to Societal Goals.* New York, N.Y.: Carnegie Corporation of New York.

Chen, P. 1992. The National Institutes of Health and its interactions with industry. In: *Biomedical Research: Collaboration and Conflict of Interest.* Porter and Malone, eds. Baltimore, Md.: The Johns Hopkins University Press, pp. 199–221.

Cole, J. R. 1993. Balancing acts: Dilemmas of choice facing research universities. *Daedalus* (Fall):1–36. Cambridge, Mass.: The American Academy of Arts and Sciences.

Committee on Small Business; Subcommittee on Business Opportunities, Regulation, and Energy; U.S. House of Representatives. 1993a. Statement of J. L. Wagner and M. E. Gluck, Office of Technology Assessment. March 11. Washington, D.C.: U.S. Government Printing Office.

Committee on Small Business; Subcommittee on Business Opportunities, Regulation, and Energy; U.S. House of Representatives. 1993b. Statement of W. A. Peck, Association of American Medical Colleges. June 17. Washington, D.C.: U.S. Government Printing Office.

Ernst and Young, 1993. *Biotech 94: Long-Term Value, Short-Term Hurdles.* San Francisco: Ernst and Young.

Feller, I. 1990. Universities as engines of R&D-based economic growth: They think they can. *Research Policy* 19:335–348.

Foote, S. B. 1992. *Managing the Medical Arms Race: Public Policy and Medical Device Innovation.* Berkeley, Calif.: University of California Press.

Gelijns, A. C. 1991. *Innovation in Clinical Practice*. Washington, D.C.: National Academy Press.

Gelijns, A. C. and N. Rosenberg. Forthcoming. Medical device innovation: Opportunities and barriers for small firms. Washington, D.C.: National Academy Press.

Ginzberg, E., and Dutka, A. B. 1989. The Financing of Biomedical Research. Baltimore, Md.: The Johns Hopkins University Press.

Health Care Technology Institute. 1994. *Insight: Variation in Research and Development Spending Within the Medical Technology Industry*. Alexandria, Va.: Health Care Technology Institute.

Hunnewell, S. 1994. The medical-industrial complex. *Harvard Magazine* (January-February):34–37.

Institute of Medicine (IOM). 1989. *Government and Industry Collaboration in Biomedical Research and Education*. Washington, D.C.: National Academy Press.

IOM. 1990. *Funding for Health Sciences Research: A Strategy to Restore the Balance*. Washington, D.C.: National Academy Press.

Laubach, G. 1994. Perspective on Academic Health Centers. *Health Affairs* (Summer):194–196.

Littell, C. L. 1994. Datawatch. Innovation in medical technology: Reading the indicators. *Health Affairs* (Summer):226–235.

National Academy of Sciences (NAS). 1986. *New Alliances and Partnerships in American Science and Engineering*. Washington, D.C.: National Academy Press.

NAS. 1991. *Industrial Perspectives on Innovation and Interactions with Universities*. Washington, D.C.: National Academy Press.

NAS. 1992. *Future National Research Policies within Industrialized Nations*. Washington, D.C.: National Academy Press.

National Science Board. 1993. *Science and Engineering Indicators—1993*. Pub. no. NSB-93-1. Washington, D.C.: U.S. Government Printing Office.

National Science Commission. 1992. *A Foundation for the 21st Century: A Progressive Framework for the National Science Foundation*. Washington, D.C.: National Science Commission.

Office of Science and Technology Policy. 1994. *Science in the National Interest*. Washington, D.C.

Pharmaceutical Manufacturers Association (PMA). 1993a. *Biotechnology Medicines in Development*. Washington, D.C.: Pharmaceutical Manufacturers Association.

PMA. 1993b. PMA Annual Survey Report: Trends in U.S. Pharmaceutical Sales and R&D. Washington, D.C.: Pharmaceutical Manufacturers Association.

Read, J. L., and Lee, Jr., K. B. 1994. Datawatch. Health care innovation: Progress report and focus on biotechnology. *Health Affairs* (Summer):215–225.

Robinson, B. 1994. Promises, promises. *Technology Transfer Business* (Winter):35–39.

Rosenberg, N., and Nelson, R. R. 1994. American Universities and Technical Advance in Industry. *Research Policy* 23:223–348.

Technology Transfer Business. 1994. SBIR accolades. (Winter):6.

U.S. Department of Health and Human Services (U.S. DHHS). 1993. *NIH Data Book 1993*. Pub. no. 93-1261. Washington, D.C.: U.S. Government Printing Office.

U.S. Department of Commerce. 1993. *U.S. Industrial Outlook 1993*. Washington, D.C.: U.S. Government Printing Office.

U.S. Department of Commerce. 1994. *U.S. Industrial Outlook 1994*. Washington, D.C. : U.S. Government Printing Office.

Weisbrod, B. A. 1994. The nature of technological change: Incentives matter! In: Institute of Medicine. *Medical Innovation at the Crossroads*, vol. 4. *Adopting New Medical Technology*. A. C. Gelijns and H. V. Dawkins, eds. Washington, D.C.: National Academy Press, pp. 8-48.

PART II

Medical Device Innovation

3
Physicians and Physicists: The Interdisciplinary Introduction of the Laser to Medicine

JOANNE SPETZ

The laser was heralded by professionals and the press, even before the first one was built in 1960. Although it was initially unclear to researchers what the laser's uses might be, there was much excitement in both the creation of the laser and the subsequent development of applications. The laser's potential in surgery was envisioned almost immediately by some of its developers owing to its ability to burn through materials; still, it is surprising that only one year after the laser's invention, it was used by an ophthalmologist to repair a retina. Most medical doctors are not educated in the principles of quantum physics, nor are physicists and engineers fully trained in the biological sciences. What institutions and relationships resulted in the development of the laser photocoagulator? The answer to this question lies in the story of the laser's development.

Scientists from many disciplines became involved in laser research in the 1960s; the laser was studied for applications in measurement, industrial production, spectroscopy, weaponry, and medicine. Such widespread interest in the laser largely resulted from the fact that the laser's creation was an interdisciplinary enterprise. The invention of the laser required the collaboration of physicists and engineers, most of which occurred in private companies. The subsequent development of laser applications followed this pattern of interdisciplinary research. The willingness of private industry to aggressively organize relationships between scientists and engineers led to the rapid introduction of the laser to medicine. By understanding the nature of these relationships and the factors that influenced them, we might better understand how new medical technologies are conceived and created.

THE LASER'S INVENTION

The demonstration of a working ruby laser by Theodore Maiman at Hughes Aircraft Corporation (see Maiman, 1960) was the culmination of over a decade of research in the stimulation of radiation, which began early in this century. In 1916, Albert Einstein laid the foundation for the invention of the laser and its predecessor, the maser, in a proof of Planck's law of radiation.[1] In 1900 the German physicist Max Planck had proposed a formula relating atoms to the spontaneous emission of electromagnetic energy. Einstein sought to relate Planck's proof to his own theories of quantum mechanics; he suggested that photon emission could be stimulated, not just spontaneously produced (see the technical appendix for a detailed explanation of laser theory). Einstein's proposal was ignored, however, until after World War II.

During World War II, several laboratories were established to develop radar. The most prominent laboratories were the Massachusetts Institute of Technology (MIT) Radiation Laboratory and the Columbia University Radiation Laboratory in the physics department. These research sites were enormously successful, and in 1946 the Joint Services Electronics Program (JSEP) was established to continue laboratory funding in peacetime. The main recipients of JSEP funds were MIT and Columbia University, and JSEP founded laboratories at Harvard in 1946 and Stanford in 1947. A variety of military projects were funded at these laboratories; one of the beneficiaries of JSEP was Charles Townes of Columbia University.

Townes had worked on radar bombing systems at Bell Laboratories in New Jersey during World War II and was a founding father of molecular and millimeter-wave spectroscopy. He became deeply involved in spectroscopy after the war, and military experts thought his work could be used in radar. Prior research of the electromagnetic spectrum had been sequential; the longest waves (electric current) were studied first, followed by shorter radio waves and then microwaves. It seemed logical to physicists to continue this pattern of development, so many projects sought to conquer waves of millimeter length. Waves with a higher frequency would be more compact than radar waves and had the potential to provide greater secrecy in communication. In 1950, the U.S. Office of Naval Research asked Townes to organize the Advisory Committee on Millimeter Wave Generation. The following year, while in Washington, D.C., to attend this committee meeting, Townes was inspired with an idea while sitting on a park bench. He thought that an oscillator made with deuterated ammonia ($ND3$) might cause the emission and amplification of microwaves (10^{-3} to 1 meter wavelengths).[2]

---

[1]Albert Einstein, *Mitt. Phys. Ges.*, 16(18):47, Zurich, 1916. An English translation is in B. L. van der Waerden, ed., *Sources of Quantum Mechanics*. Amsterdam: North-Holland, 1967.

[2]This idea clearly had its roots in Einstein's theory that electromagnetic emissions could be stimulated.

Townes' colleagues were skeptical of this idea and argued that a high-frequency emission could not result from Townes' device. Despite the lukewarm reception of his ideas, Townes began work on an oscillator with Herbert J. Zeiger, a postdoctoral student, and James P. Gordon, a doctoral candidate, in the fall of 1951.

Zeiger and Gordon began to build what Townes later called a MASER— Microwave Amplification by Stimulated Emission of Radiation—in 1952. Construction was supported by the Army Signal Corps, the U.S. Air Force, and the Office of Naval Research through JSEP. Zeiger left the project in February 1953 when his postdoctoral appointment ended but Gordon continued working with Townes. They demonstrated the amplification of microwaves by the end of the year and, in April 1954, generated a microwave oscillation with a power output of 0.01 microwatt. An explosion of MASER (now "maser") research followed their announcement.

Part of Townes' success with the maser can be attributed to his education as an electrical engineer. His approach to his work involved a combination of physics theory and engineering application. Once he was convinced that a maser could work, he focused on the task of engineering a device to prove his theory. Townes' association with several corporations through the Carbide and Carbon Chemicals Corporation Post-graduate Fellows Program at Columbia's Radiation Laboratory was also a result of his engineering background. This was one of the ways he kept abreast of the commercial possibilities of his research. He was aware that the maser could prove useful in many industrial and military applications.

Following the invention of the maser, many researchers began to develop applications for it. Government agencies explored several uses for the maser. Because a very narrow band of wavelengths are emitted by a maser, the maser was an attractive candidate for measurement applications such as a frequency standard or an atomic clock.[3] Private companies, especially those with close ties to the military, sought to reap profit from Townes' invention. The military was interested in having a portable generator of a frequency standard for guided missiles and the Army Signal Corps Engineering Laboratory provided funding to the Jet Propulsion Laboratory in Pasadena, California, to research this.[4] Hughes Aircraft's Research and Development Laboratory hired the former chief of the Microwave Standards Section of the National Bureau of Standards to improve Hughes' competitiveness for military contracts.

A result of maser research was a closer relationship between engineering and

---

[3]The trait of a narrow band of wavelengths being emitted is often called the "pureness" of the frequency of the maser.

[4]Airborne Instruments Laboratory, a small company for which Townes consulted, also received an Air Force contract in 1955 to study the same thing. This duplication of projects by different divisions of the military was typical during the 1950s.

physics. Private companies hired both engineers and physicists for their new millimeter-wave research laboratories and as engineers entered the field they made significant contributions in the development of maser systems. Because the maser made understanding quantum mechanics necessary for electrical engineering, engineering curricula were altered throughout the United States in the late 1950s. Schools decided to diversify engineering education and to increase the scientific content of course work. Older graduate students and professors had to learn new material to remain at the forefront of engineering.[5] Interdisciplinary educations and collaborations were key to the inventions of both the maser and the laser and to the development of applications for them.

After conquering the emission of waves in the radio and microwave spectra, many scientists viewed the infrared region (10^{-6} to 10^{-3} meters) as the next step. Millimeter and submillimeter waves became the focus of radio engineering research in the late 1950s. Many ideas came from the maser principle and proposals for tackling this region were issued by universities, private laboratories, and Department of Defense-sponsored laboratories. At the end of the summer of 1957, Townes began a serious study of the infrared maser. As he developed ideas, he leapt over the infrared frequencies and focused on visible light (4×10^{-7} to 7×10^{-7} meter wavelengths). He began to create design ideas for an "optical maser" and contacted Arthur Schawlow of Bell Labs, where Townes was a consultant.[6] They agreed to work together and Bell Labs filed a patent application for their optical maser proposal a year later. Schawlow and Townes sent a manuscript of their theoretical calculations to *Physics Review*, which published their paper that year (Schawlow and Townes, 1958).

At the same time that Townes began work with Schawlow, Townes met R. Gordon Gould, a graduate student at Columbia University. Gould was working on a doctoral thesis on the energy level of excited thallium and was familiar with the parallel reflecting plates called Fabry-Perot etalons which Schawlow envisioned using for the optical maser. Gould and Townes had conversations on the general subject of radiation emission and Gould made notes about his ideas for a LASER (Light Amplification by Stimulated Emission of Radiation) in November 1957 and had them notarized.[7] His notes included possible applications for a laser, such as spectrometry, interferometry, radar, and nuclear fusion. In March 1958 he took a job at Technical Research Group (TRG) without finishing his dissertation with the agreement that any inventions he had dated before his hiring date would remain his property. In July of that year, TRG gave Gould free time to work on his doctoral thesis. Gould worked on the laser instead.

He wrote detailed plans for the creation of such a device and filed a patent application in April 1959. Bell Labs won the patent in 1960 and were then

---

5A discussion of these changes can be found in Bromberg (1991), pp. 42–43.
6Schawlow was a close professional colleague and was Townes' brother-in-law.
7"Laser" became the popular term for optical masers.

challenged by TRG and Gould. This conflict continued for several years, with Bell as the ultimate victor.[8]

Meanwhile, after the publication of the Schawlow and Townes (1958) paper on the optical maser, a race had begun to construct the first working laser. At least six laboratories, most in private companies, were involved in this research: Columbia University, Bell Labs, TRG, IBM, Hughes, and American Optical Corporation. The private companies expected a laser to have many applications, although there was little substantial discussion of uses for the laser until after its invention.

The first "lasing" of a substance was achieved by Theodore Maiman at Hughes on May 16, 1960, with a ruby crystal laser small enough to hold with one hand. His breakthrough was published in *Nature* in July of that year (Maiman, 1960) and before the year ended three other materials were lased. The new laser exhibited several previously unknown physical effects, and it was clear to scientists that much research could be done about and with the laser. The desire to develop applications for this invention led to a flurry of research, primarily by private-sector companies. Firms hoped to obtain patents for laser uses and to win military contracts before their competitors did. It is estimated that 400 to 500 laboratories were studying the laser in the early 1960s. Laser manufacturers proposed laser applications that would expand their markets: Bell Labs studied optical communications, Martin-Marietta worked on laser target designators, and Hughes Aircraft designed optical radars.

In 1963, the *Proceedings of the Institute of Electronics and Electrical Engineers* contained an article about the laser that reviewed anticipated applications, including medical, industrial, photographic, scientific, and communications uses (*Proceedings of the IEEE*, 1963). The laser was also celebrated in the popular press. *Time*, *U.S. News and World Report*, and the *Wall Street Journal* published articles in the early 1960s about the laser's promise for the future. In 1963 the *Wall Street Journal* predicted that the laser could reach $1 billion in sales by 1973 (cited in Bromberg, 1991). Such proclamations resulted in a rush of venture capital to the new laser industry. Established firms and new companies marketed commercial lasers, with the first ones being sold in 1961. By 1963, about 20 firms were selling lasers. While the sales volume was low, the availability of lasers encouraged research throughout the country.

It was during this early heyday of laser development that medical uses were envisioned and research began in New York and California. This research was a continuation of two trends in medical research: that of photocoagulation and that of studying the dangers of radiation. Relationships between medical doctors and physicists led to the introduction of the laser to these trends and the resultant production of the first medical laser device, the laser photocoagulator.

---

[8]Details of this conflict are available in many accounts of the development of the laser, including Bromberg (1991), pp. 69–75.

PHOTOCOAGULATION

Medical research with the laser was largely the result of a connection between the ongoing work of ophthalmologists and the laser's providing a powerful light source. In 1954 a German ophthalmologist, Gerd Meyer-Schwickerath, introduced photocoagulation to the treatment of retinal disease (see Meyer-Schwickerath, 1967, 1973). He created a device that concentrated the sun's light to a small focal point and used this light energy to create a lesion in the retina. These lesions served as welds to prevent retinal detachment which was then the leading cause of blindness despite the existence of this procedure. Before Meyer-Schwickerath's discovery, coagulation of the retina required the ophthalmologist to either apply energy on the surface of the eye with a diathermy machine or turn the eye around after loosening muscles to bore a hole in the sclera and use an inflammatory material such as lye to create an adhesion. This procedure required an inpatient hospital stay and significant recuperation time and was, as Dr. Francis L'Esperance commented, "really barbaric" (see Hecht, 1986).

In the mid-1950s, xenon high-pressure arc lamps became available. They had been developed by the American Optical Corporation in Southbridge, Massachusetts, for a movie producer and were so bright that the light would coagulate the back of the eye if a person looked at it. Zeiss Laboratories in Oberlochen, Germany, began to manufacture a photocoagulator with the xenon lamp. The first three Zeiss coagulators arrived in the United States in 1959. The recipients included the Edward S. Harkness Eye Institute at Columbia-Presbyterian Medical Center in New York and the Stanford University Medical Center.

The Zeiss photocoagulator was a great advance in the treatment of retinal disease but it had several disadvantages. Zeiss treatment requires the dilation of the pupil, and the lesions produced by the Zeiss are large since the light beams emitted are wide. Patients experience pain during the half-second treatment because, as Dr. Milton Flocks of Stanford University explained, "in half a second . . . the iris contracts and comes down hard, and that hurts" (personal communication, Milton Flocks, March 20, 1992). Ophthalmologists wanted a better light source for photocoagulation, and several companies experimented with improved lamps.

Photocoagulation was highly publicized, so it is not surprising that some developers of the laser recognized that their invention might provide an appropriate light source for ophthalmological treatment. Early demonstrations of the laser by Schawlow included one with a dark balloon inside a clear balloon. When he aimed the laser at the pair the light passed through the clear balloon and popped the dark one.[9] He later commented that it was obvious that "once you

---

[9]Light is absorbed differently by differently colored materials, depending on the wavelength of light. The ruby laser has a wavelength of 694 nanometers, which is absorbed by darker materials, such as a retina.

had a brighter light, it was worth trying" for retinal surgery (reported in Hecht, 1992). Townes also recognized this potential in ophthalmology and wrote a paper in the early 1960s about possible medical and biological uses of the laser (Townes, 1962). But before the laser was considered for therapeutic work, researchers studied the potential danger of the laser to the eye.

FEAR OF INJURY

The physicists and engineers who invented and worked with the laser recognized its danger immediately. Accounts of retinal damage caused by staring at eclipses were reported by Plato and, more recently, many people had experienced retinal burns from watching the nuclear explosions at Hiroshima and Nagasaki. When doctors began treating vision-impaired residents of Japan they conducted systematic research on flash burns of the retina. Among these researchers were William Ham, Jr., and his associates at the Medical College of Virginia. His group, with support from the Defense Atomic Support Agency, studied flash burns on rabbit retinae in the late 1950s (Ham, Jr., et al., 1963). This research alerted ophthalmologists to the dangers of powerful light sources and resulted in government sponsorship of studies of the laser's effects. The government was interested both in ensuring the safety of scientists and technicians and in developing a laser weapon.

The first papers about the laser's risks appeared in *Science* on November 10, 1961. Two articles were published, one by Leonard Solon, Raphael Aronson, and Gordon Gould of TRG (Solon et al., 1961) and the other by Milton M. Zaret and his associates at the New York University Medical Center (Zaret et al., 1961). Zaret served as a medical consultant to TRG and Bell Labs and was pursuing two careers: one as an ophthalmologist and one as a researcher on the effects of radiation on humans. His primary interest was (and is) the relationship between nonionized radiation and cancer, and he had been a consultant to the military for radar and microwave research. His positions at TRG and Bell required that he examine the employees of these companies to determine what levels of exposure workers had to radiation. Because he communicated directly with the companies' researchers, he heard about new and ongoing research projects. He became aware of laser research in 1959 and understood the potential optical effects of a laser; he also understood the risk of injury the laser posed, especially to the eye. Zaret had "more than a casual knowledge of physics" (personal communication, Milton M. Zaret, May 1, 1992). He had been trained as an engineer during his military service in World War II and had written a graduate chemistry thesis on the structure of the atom, a subject that would now be in the realm of atomic physics. This interdisciplinary scientific education enabled him to fully understand the laser and its effects on human tissue; every ophthalmologist who developed laser photocoagulation systems in the early 1960s had a similarly strong knowledge of physics.

Immediately after Maiman's announcement (Maiman, 1960), Zaret began to study the ruby laser's effects on human tissue. He was able to access laser equipment because of his contact with Bell Labs and TRG. He studied the lesions induced on a rabbit's retina and iris and determined that the ruby laser could cause significant damage to the human eye. The first paper on his findings was published in *Science* in 1961 (Zaret et al., 1961). He also recognized that this damage could be therapeutic, as photocoagulation. The accompanying article by Solon and his colleagues (1961) contained theoretical calculations of the laser's effect on the retina. Solon concluded that the ruby laser had the energy density of viewing the sun directly for 30 seconds, which is six times the density needed to burn the retina. The implication of these publications was that the laser presented a physical risk and that more research was needed to understand the laser's effects on humans. Zaret continued to study this throughout the 1960s (see Zaret et al., 1962, 1963).

Further quantitative research was conducted by Ham and his associates in the mid-1960s. Their work was funded by the U.S. Army Medical Research and Development Command, the Office of the Surgeon General, and the Defense Atomic Support Agency. They noted in a 1963 paper that there was a "recognized need to study the biological effect of lasers, especially due to the ocular hazard of retinal burns" (Ham et al., 1963). Ham's group built a ruby laser and identified thresholds for irreversible injury. The conclusion was that the ruby laser produced four levels of short-term damage to the retina: (1) blanching of the retina, (2) cavitation or bubble formation, (3) breakthrough of the vitreous, and (4) hemorrhage in addition to the first three effects. While the results of Zaret's and Ham's research might have been viewed pessimistically by those with little knowledge of medicine, the identification and description of the dangers of the laser were necessary to facilitate its development as a therapeutic tool.

POTENTIAL IN OPHTHALMOLOGY

Two groups of researchers independently began work with the laser as a therapeutic device at roughly the same time. The first group to commence experimentation was that of Dr. Charles J. Campbell of the Institute of Ophthalmology at Columbia-Presbyterian Medical Center in Manhattan and Dr. Charles Koester of the above-mentioned American Optical Corporation in Southbridge, Massachusetts. The other group was based at Stanford University and was headed by Drs. Milton Flocks and Christian Zweng. Flocks was a half-time researcher on the clinical faculty at Stanford and Zweng was a practicing ophthalmologist at the Palo Alto Medical Foundation while holding a faculty position. They collaborated with Dr. Narinder Kapany, a physicist who founded Optics Technology, Incorporated, in 1960.

These groups were similar in both their composition and their research. Both the New York and the California group were comprised of researchers from private industry and from academic medical centers. The two companies involved, American Optical and Optics Technology, developed relationships with medical researchers in order to design and test new medical devices. The ophthalmologists did not have the means to create the laser photocoagulator without the resources of private industry, but both Charles Campbell and Milton Flocks had educations that enabled them to understand the laser. Campbell had earned a master's degree in optics from the Institute of Optics of the University of Rochester before beginning his residency in ophthalmology (personal communication, Charles Koester, April 29, 1993). Flocks had taken a graduate course in atomic physics while in college. He also had studied pathology under a Heed Fellowship at the Armed Forces Institute of Pathology before he moved to California. Lastly, Charles Campbell, Milton Flocks, and Christian Zweng had conducted research with the Zeiss photocoagulators their medical centers received in 1959.

American Optical established its laser research program in 1959 by hiring Elias Snitzer. Snitzer was a specialist in fiber optics and had developed military electro-optics in the 1950s. Shortly after Maiman's announcement of the ruby laser in 1960, Snitzer constructed one for his own experimentation. Charles Koester was simultaneously developing an improved photocoagulator with a mercury arc lamp. Since Snitzer knew of Koester's project, he realized that the laser had potential for photocoagulation. Sometime in late 1960, Snitzer asked Koester if the ruby laser would be a suitable light source. Koester made some calculations based on the energy and wavelength of the laser and "concluded it made sense" (see Bromberg, 1984). American Optical started a research program on laser photocoagulation before the end of 1960.

Koester contacted Charles Campbell, then a medical consultant for American Optical, for a medical opinion and to conduct clinical experiments. In the fall of 1961 they used a prototype ruby laser photocoagulator on a patient for the first time, destroying a retinal tumor. The results of this experiment were publicized in a press release which, at the request of Dr. Campbell, named only Dr. Koester. Articles were published in the *New York Times* and the *Wall Street Journal* on December 22, 1961. In the spring of 1962, Koester, Snitzer, and Campbell presented a paper on their work at a meeting of the Optical Society of America (Koester et al., 1962). Milton Zaret also discussed his rabbit experiments at the meeting (Zaret et al., 1962). Koester and Campbell were unaware of Zaret's work until the Optical Society of America meeting. They also did not know that Milton Flocks and Christian Zweng were in the early stages of their laser research in 1961.

Flocks and Zweng had written one paper together before attending a conference in 1955 at which Gerd Meyer-Schwickerath described the Zeiss photocoagulator. After hearing Meyer-Schwickerath's presentation, Zweng and Flocks applied for and received a grant from the National Institutes of Health to obtain a Zeiss instrument. Zweng and Flocks' research with the photo-coagulator was publicized throughout the San Francisco area.

In 1962 a Stanford scientist showed Flocks a "little ruby laser the size of a pencil" and told Flocks it could produce more light than the Zeiss instrument (personal communication, Milton Flocks, March 20, 1992). According to Flocks, the scientist who took the laser to the medical school was unaware of other medical research involving the laser. Shortly after this meeting, Flocks and Zweng contacted someone in the physics department at Stanford who built a ruby laser for them to conduct preliminary research. Zweng also consulted with Milton Zaret, as Zaret was assisting several researchers in the development of laser research laboratories. Zweng and Flocks began working with rabbits, monkeys, and cats and published the results of their research on a rabbit and a cat in July 1963. Flocks and Zweng used the instrument on a human for the first time in August 1963 (Kapany et al., 1963; Zweng et al., 1964).

By 1964 a large amount of research had been conducted by the California and New York groups (see, for example, Campbell et al., 1963a,b; Koester et al., 1962; Zweng and Flocks, 1965). Their research became known to the medical community primarily through conferences and publications. Koester and Campbell and Milton Zaret had presented papers at the aforementioned Optical Society of America meeting in the spring of 1962. Campbell presented a paper on laser coagulation at the Southeastern Section meeting of the American Association for Research in Ophthalmology (AARO) in March of that year. At the AARO meeting, Campbell stated that their study "demonstrates clearly that a laser photocoagulator has potential as a safe clinical device." At the American Medical Association meeting of June 1964, Flocks and Zweng described 25 patients who had been treated exclusively with the ruby laser. The reaction from the medical community was strong; as Flocks recalls, "All these doctors didn't even know what a laser was. They'd never heard the word, most of them . . . and after that [the presentation at the conference] it went like wildfire." Still, a voice of caution remained in the medical profession. After Flocks and Zweng's presentation, Milton Zaret rose to discuss their paper and stated that it was irresponsible of them to use the laser on human subjects given that they didn't know the laser's long-term effects. Zaret also expressed concern about the danger of the laser to the laser operator and assistant, since these people would be exposed to its radiation repeatedly. Since much of Zaret's other research was focused on the long-term effects of radiation, his concerns were well-founded. Much more research was needed before the laser would be accepted by ophthalmologists.

PHOTOCOAGULATORS AND THE PRIVATE SECTOR

After the laser's initial clinical trials by Flocks and Zweng and by Campbell, research on photocoagulation took a new form. The indications for and limitations of laser photocoagulation needed determination, as it was clear that the technique could be valuable to the treatment of eye disease. More importantly, sophisticated equipment was needed to provide doctors with greater control over the beam. Medical doctors actively collaborated with laser manufacturers to design equipment specifically for medical use; American Optical sponsored the first use of a laser photocoagulator on a human subject and subsequently began to develop a commercial device, and Milton Flocks and Christian Zweng began work with Optics Technology shortly after their first experiments with the laser photocoagulator. Zweng also co-authored the first book on laser photocoagulation in 1969 (see Zweng et al., 1969).

As mentioned earlier, Optics Technology, Incorporated, was founded in 1960 by Narinder Kapany, a physicist educated in India. Kapany is "generally acknowledged to be the originator of fiber optics" (*Laser Focus*, 1967). His doctoral thesis sought to prove that one could send an image through fibers much as one could deliver other electronic signals; it laid the groundwork for the development of the fiberoptic endoscope. He used Optics Technology as a vehicle for research on the application of new technologies.[10]

Who initiated the collaboration between Drs. Zweng and Flocks and Dr. Kapany is unclear. Flocks and Zweng, after their initial research on rabbits, found that the laser they had received from the physics department was not ideal. The physics department was unable to assist them in producing better equipment, so they sought a private laser supplier. In 1961 Kapany received a grant from the National Institutes of Health (the first given to a private company) titled "Applications of Modern Optics in Medicine." He cultivated relationships with cardiologists, gastroenterologists, proctologists, radiologists, and ophthalmologists. Flocks and Zweng were among those who received lasers from and consulted with Kapany.

According to Kapany, a project was planned to test laser interaction with human tissue (see Cunningham, 1986; personal communication, Narinder Kapany, May 14, 1992). Kapany asked an employee, Dr. Ig Liu, to build a laser for this project. A device composed of a steel tube with a ruby rod and flashlamps was suggested, and when Liu showed Kapany the product Kapany immediately suggested that an ophthalmic head be added to it. This equipment was the basis for Optics Technology's photocoagulator. Zweng, Flocks, and scientists at Optics Technology defined their specifications: constant energy output, protection of the laser operator, viewing capability, easy aiming, the ability to create a useful lesion, variation in the laser pulse, maneuverability of the instrument, and the ability to change the size of the focal point of the beam. By early 1963 a prototype had been developed, and it may have been this photocoagulator that Zweng and Flocks used on their first human subject.

Kapany made a public announcement of this experimental photocoagulator and selected 20 ophthalmologists to purchase the instrument and provide clinical data to Optics Technology. As the success of laser treatment became apparent to

---

[10]Arthur Schawlow was on the board of directors of Optics Technology.

the medical community, Optics Technology was able to sell many photocoagulation devices. American Optical's photocoagulator reached the marketplace in late 1963. Campbell and Koester developed the device with funding from the National Institute of Neurological Diseases and Blindness and the U.S. Public Health Service. Their device was more sophisticated and more expensive than that of Optics Technology (personal communication, Charles Koester, April 29, 1993) and sold at the rate of about a dozen per year. According to Kapany, Optics Technology and American Optical "didn't have any competitors until almost the year 1968 when Coherent Radiation came out with an argon photocoagulator" (reported in Cunningham, 1986).

The argon laser was invented in 1964 and within a year researchers used this light source for photocoagulation. The laser was a great improvement over the Zeiss instrument in many cases, especially since the laser's brief exposure time reduced pain and its monochromatic light was more easily controlled than white light. Patients could be treated on an outpatient basis and no anesthesia was needed. Still, the ruby laser photocoagulator had several disadvantages and was not used for some retinal disorders. The major complaints against the ruby laser were that the laser pulsed in a slightly irregular fashion, the intensity of the output was difficult to control, and the beam diameter varied (Campbell et al., 1963). A laser that could create similar lesions in the eye without these disadvantages was desired and was found in the argon laser.

In early 1965 Dr. Francis L'Esperance of the Columbia-Presbyterian Medical Center presented his first paper on treating diabetic retinopathy (then the leading cause of blindness in people 20 to 64 years old) with a ruby laser at a conference in New York. L'Esperance, like Zaret, Flocks, and Campbell, had a remarkably strong knowledge of physics; he says he "had taken every physics and chemistry course at Dartmouth College" (reported in Hecht, 1986). He became interested in laser photocoagulation after hearing about the early research of Flocks, Zweng, and Campbell. L'Esperance bought the third ruby laser made by Optics Technology for $5,500 in 1963 and began research on humans the following year. In his 1965 presentation on the ruby laser, L'Esperance noted that doctors needed a blue-green laser since its wavelength would be likely to produce therapeutic lesions. In the discussion following the presentation, Flocks said he had just seen an argon laser in a Palo Alto company's research laboratory (personal communication, Milton Flocks, March 20, 1992).

Shortly after the 1965 conference, L'Esperance learned from a patient that Bell Laboratories had developed a blue-green laser. L'Esperance began placing phone calls immediately. He contacted Eugene Gordon and Edward Labuda of Bell Labs and had "a very stiff meeting" at which Gordon and Labuda sought to determine the specifications L'Esperance wanted (reported in Hecht, 1986). L'Esperance could not provide such information; since the argon laser was new, L'Esperance had no sense of its effects on the eye. The three men met several more times, but Gordon and Labuda were reluctant to pursue a project with

L'Esperance because Bell Labs' charter is for auditory, not visual, devices. They found an excuse to work on optical applications when they saw someone working on a prototype picturephone; at that point "things started changing" (Hecht, 1986). As with the development of the ruby laser, the collaboration of academic and private-sector researchers proved fruitful.

Gordon loaned L'Esperance several laser discharge tubes and L'Esperance began to determine what power levels were necessary for successful photocoagulation. Raytheon developed the most powerful argon ion laser in existence for L'Esperance's work and in early 1966 studies were initiated on animals. The first human was treated with the argon laser in February 1968, at which time L'Esperance decided to design a device for ophthalmological clinics. He called the John A. Hartford Foundation of New York, a private foundation that provides funding for medical research. After hearing L'Esperance's description of the project, the director of the foundation replied, "Forget all the preliminary stuff. All I want is the budget" (quoted in Hecht, 1986). L'Esperance received $287,000 to begin work with Bell Labs in 1968.[11]

In 1968 and 1969, with Gordon and Labuda, L'Esperance developed three delivery systems for ophthalmologists. A fourth system was created in association with the American Optical Corporation. An indirect delivery device and an articulated-arm manipulator that allowed one to hold the laser like a scalpel were among the new instruments. L'Esperance published the designs so they went into the public domain and tested them clinically with Dr. Felix Shiffman[12] (see L'Esperance, 1968, 1973; L'Esperance et al., 1969). The argon laser proved superior to the ruby laser and, according to Flocks, "as soon as the argon was developed, everything else disappeared." In 1969, Coherent Incorporated decided to produce and market the Bell designs, which are still the standard for photocoagulators.

Coherent's profitable sales of the argon laser were not surprising to those working on laser photocoagulation. First, lasers were clearly superior to conventional white light sources for photocoagulation. Further, most ophthalmological laser researchers, according to Elias Snitzer, "were aware of the fact that it was necessary to shift the wavelength into the green" (reported in Bromberg, 1984). American Optical did not pursue the argon coagulator because they did not have a research program on argon lasers in place (personal communication, Charles Koester, April 29, 1993) and because the ruby laser photocoagulator had not been profitable (Bromberg, 1984). Optics Technology also did not design an argon device, leaving the market completely available to Coherent.

---

[11]Zweng and Flocks also applied for a grant from the Hartford Foundation. Their request was submitted after L'Esperance's, and they were informed that the foundation had just given a grant for the same thing to Dr. L'Esperance.

[12]When asked why he didn't patent these designs, L'Esperance responded, "Doctors didn't do that; we wanted to get potential manufacturers interested and people treated" (reported in Hecht, 1986).

By 1971, Christian Zweng and other doctors were teaching argon laser photocoagulation courses throughout the United States. Diabetic retinopathy was no longer a major threat to eyesight and, thus far, there have been no systemic negative effects of laser treatment in ophthalmology. The laser is used by ophthalmologists for glaucoma treatment, retinal reattachment, and the ablation of tumors. As Leon Goldman noted in *Laser Focus*, (1967), "eye surgery . . . is now almost accepted as routine by nearly everybody." In 1990, 95 percent of ophthalmologists surveyed by Arthur D. Little, Inc., agreed that they "recognize the laser as a legitimate medical tool and use it when it is the superior method of treatment" (Arthur D. Little Decision Resources, Inc., 1989; Halter, 1985). Research of the laser's effects on other parts of the body has progressed more slowly than ophthalmological research owing to the difficulty of working with more complex tissue structures. What advancement has occurred is not strictly the result of ophthalmology's success being transferred to other specialties; significant research was performed by doctors in other fields in the early 1960s.

MORE EARLY MEDICAL LASER RESEARCH

In 1986, John L. Ratz wrote in the introduction to a textbook on lasers in nonophthalmological medicine that "the birth of laser medicine in the early 1960s was largely due to the hard work and persistence of Leon Goldman, M.D." (Ratz, 1986). Given the breadth of work conducted and supervised by Goldman at the University of Cincinnati, this statement is probably not an exaggeration. He was the first person to use the ruby laser in dermatology and has been dubbed the "father of lasers in medicine and surgery" by the medical profession.[13] His studies involved almost every laser developed and most parts of the human (and animal) body. Because Goldman studied a wide range of biologic effects, many medical specialties benefited from his lifelong work.

Goldman's laser research began in 1962 when the Occupational Health Division of the U.S. Public Health Service and the Hartford Foundation provided funding to the department of dermatology at the University of Cincinnati to establish a medical laser laboratory. The laboratory was placed under Dr. Goldman's leadership at the Cincinnati General Hospital. According to Milton Zaret, Goldman consulted Zaret for assistance in the early stages of the laboratory's development (personal communication, Milton M. Zaret, May 1, 1992). The purpose of the laser laboratory was "to study the occupational hazards of the laser . . . primarily the dangers to physicists and technicians in laser laboratories."[14]

This laboratory's early work focused on laser safety, particularly the proper

---

[13]This statement has been made by Choy (1988), Ratz (1986), and others.
[14]Dr. Goldman described this project and other work in *Laser Focus* (March 1967).

construction of facilities and the protection of workers. Goldman's first published medical study appeared in the *Journal of Investigative Dermatology* in January 1963 (Goldman et al., 1963a). He presented a summary of the effects of the laser on white and black skin and rabbit eyes. The most significant finding was that the ruby laser's effect on tissue depends on the skin's melanin content and degree of vascularization; darker-colored tissues exhibit more damage than light-colored tissue. Goldman concluded his paper by noting that he was studying the laser's effect on red cells, capillaries, pigmented nevi, basal cell carcinomas, and tattoos.

Shortly after the founding of Goldman's laser laboratory, the Hartford Foundation and the National Institutes of Health (NIH) provided him with another grant to develop an applied medical laser laboratory. The particular interest of the Hartford Foundation, NIH, and Goldman was to develop surgical instrumentation for basic research and clinical studies. By 1965 the new medical laser laboratory was considered "one of the best-equipped laser research laboratories in the U.S.A." (*Laser Focus*, 1965). It contained 10 rooms, eight lasers, and an interdisciplinary staff of 30 biologists, histologists, cytologists, physicists, and instrument design engineers.

Goldman's laboratory completed important investigations regarding the laser in hematology, cytology, protein and enzyme research, dentistry, retinal coagulation, and dermatology. Procedures for treating skin cancers and for removing tattoos and warts were developed by Goldman. Goldman supervised experiments of whether the laser produced malignancies in animals and whether the vapor resulting from laser contact with tissue was harmful. He also recognized that the transmission of laser beams through rods would be significant to medicine, and his laboratory was the first to report delivery of ruby laser beams to skin with a fiberoptic device (see Goldman et al., 1963a,b).

Much of Goldman's interest in this new, larger laboratory came from the realization that laser instrumentation for surgery was "primitive" and that "laser manufacturers are not interested in the production of equipment for medical purposes" (*Laser Focus*, 1965). Companies were reluctant to enter the medical laser market for at least three reasons: development costs were high, the laser companies were not familiar with medical buyers, and small companies could not protect their inventions from larger corporations. The solution to this reluctance was a large infusion of government money, particularly from the NIH and the military.

Early laser research was occurring in what Susan Bartlett Foote (1992) called "the heyday of federal biomedical support," and the Armed Forces became interested in using the laser as a beam weapon. Milton Flocks, Milton Zaret, and Charles Koester commented on the military's interest in identifying the threshold to damage from the laser in preparation for using it as a weapon. Flocks commented that such research "was not of much interest to me," and Milton Zaret, who received grants from the Air Force Systems Command, concurs. Military interest in the laser was not exhibited strictly through grants; in 1965 *Laser Focus* reported that the Army Missile Command at the Redstone Arsenal was developing a high-energy laser medical unit. The project reportedly began when Dr. John P. Minton of the National Cancer Institute was searching for a high-powered laser and learned that the military could provide one. Dr. James R. Dearman of Redstone called this program "the result of a unique marriage between the military and medicine" (*Laser Focus*, 1965). The U.S. government's and military's interest in the laser was beneficial to medicine resulting in a large volume of important research from government-supported projects.

Medical laser research developed an audience from the large number of medical and laser conferences in the 1960s. It was through these events that the medical profession informed laser developers of their needs. At the Boston Laser Conference in August 1964, Goldman and Zaret reported on the dangers of the laser to scientists, while Captain Martin S. Litwin of the Army Medical Research and Development Command stated that biological researchers needed continuous lasers, especially at wavelengths shorter than 5900 angstroms. The 1965 Northeast Electronics Research and Engineering Meeting included 10 papers on medical uses, including one by Goldman. The watershed event for medical research may have been the First Annual Biomedical Conference on Laser Research, organized by Dr. Paul E. McGuff of Tufts New England Medical Center, and featuring 36 talks. In 1965, Goldman began to bring his work to doctors more directly; he inquired in *Laser Focus* whether medical professionals were interested in a course on the use of lasers.

Other projects involving the laser were few in the early 1960s. Dentists began examining the laser's effect on teeth in 1964, with studies focusing on human enamel, dentin, and dental restorative materials. While this research was needed to understand the laser's effects on human tissue, it produced no immediate advances for dentistry. Marginally more successful were studies of the laser's potential in surgery (Wolbarsht, 1971).

Dr. McGuff published reports on the use of the laser in surgery in 1963. By 1964, with David Prushnell of Raytheon, he vaporized a human carcinoma that had been transplanted to a hamster. Early cancer studies were the mechanism by which the vaporization and cutting abilities of the laser became fully known. A flurry of research on laser treatments for cancer occurred in the mid-1960s, but cancer treatment studies became less common after scientists discovered that the ablation was scattering malignant cells to other sites (Bromberg, 1991).

Laser surgery equipment began to appear in the medical marketplace in 1965 with the development of microsurgical equipment by M.C. Bessis and others at the National Transfusion Center in Paris. In 1967, Laser Incorporated, a spin-off from and subsidiary of American Optical Corporation, introduced a portable surgical device designed for operating room use. Prototypes were tested on dogs at the Montefiore Hospital Medical Center in New York.

By the mid-1960s there were many types of lasers available for researchers;

the neodymium-doped yttrium-aluminum-garnet (Nd:YAG) laser had been developed in 1964 by Bell Labs, as had the carbon dioxide ($CO2$) laser in 1965. It was known that the $CO2$ laser vaporized tissue, the Nd:YAG created a coagulative necrosis within tissue, and the visible lasers (ruby, argon, etc.) served as hemostatic coagulators. Because the biological effect of a laser is dependent on the laser's wavelength, energy density, and tissue absorption, doctors needed to develop an understanding of the principles of light transmission, scatter, reflection, and absorption. Theoretically, surgeons could manipulate the laser beam's width and energy density to obtain a desired effect, but medical scientists did not understand the laser well enough to define these parameters. The determination of the indications for and best method of use of the laser has been the focus of laser research since 1965.

THE MEDICAL LASER INDUSTRY TODAY

Even over 30 years after Zaret's preliminary paper (Zaret ct al., 1961) on the laser, new medical uses for the laser are announced frequently. Current proposals include using the laser for lithotripsy (the breaking up of kidney stones), phototherapy treatment of cancer, recanalization of arteries, and Doppler-shift measurement of blood velocity (see Forrester, 1988; Hall, 1990; Ratz, 1986; Sanborn, 1988; Sliney and Wolbarsht, 1989; White, 1988). The laser is now commonly used in ophthalmology, in otolaryngology to treat benign lesions in the throat, in gynecological surgery to treat endometriosis and remove cervical dysplasia, in gastroenterology, and in dermatology (see Table 3-1), which are a few of the fields that have had either established clinical experience with the laser or randomized controlled trials (see Table 3-2). More importantly, the laser has been proven the best treatment for some indications, especially in ophthalmology (see Table 3-2). New research is made possible by an active medical technology industry in the United States, although this industry's success is often affected by forces beyond its control.

During the end of the 1960s the laser marketplace underwent significant changes. The laser shifted to mostly civilian use and the Mansfield Amendment of 1969 prohibited defense agencies from supporting basic research. NIH began to focus more on scientific research than on technological development. Most research and development received its funding from outside the public sector and entrepreneurial individuals sought venture capital for their ideas. New companies were created frequently as engineers tried to capitalize on the laser's popularity. They obtained funds from private investors but encountered many difficulties entering the medical industry due to the particularities of its institutions and regulations.

Medical device development is generally less expensive than pharmaceutical development because of the comparative simplicity of mechanical and electrical design. Medical devices, however, are less protectable by patents, making many

TABLE 3-1 Rate of Laser Penetration by Specialty,[a]
1985–1990

Specialty	1985	1988	1990
Ophthalmology	65	90	95
Otolaryngology	30	45	55
Gastroenterology	25	40	50
Obstetrics/gynecology	20	30	35
Dermatology/reconstructive surgery	15	25	35
Neurosurgery	14	20	30
Podiatry	8	20	35
Urology	7	10	25
Thoracic surgery	4	10	15
General surgery	2	5	10
Orthopedics	1	5	10
Cardiovascular surgery	0	5	10
Oncology	1	1	3
Dentistry	0	0	3

[a]Percent of physicians who "recognize the laser as a legitimate medical tool and use it when it is the superior method of treatment."

SOURCE: Arthur D. Little Decision Resources, Inc., 1989.

researchers reluctant to devote resources to the creation of a new medical tool. The Food and Drug Administration's (FDA) oversight of the licensing process of medical devices further hinders innovation. The FDA began to regulate devices stringently with the 1976 Medical Device Amendments, codifying requirements for the testing and approval of new devices (Kessler et al., 1987). Although many researchers complain about the FDA approval process, Dr. Jacob Dagan of Advanced Surgical Technologies, Inc., Dr. Leroy Sutter of Directed Energy, Inc., and Kenneth Nilsson of Cooper Lasersonics, Inc., agree that "FDA regulations have been of minimum detriment" to the success of lasers in medicine (Akerley, 1985).

Federal policies for financing health care also affect the medical laser device market. When Medicare and Medicaid were established in 1965, payments were made to doctors and hospitals on a fee-for-service basis. In 1984, the Health Care Financing Administration (HCFA, which oversees Medicare and Medicaid) established the Prospective Payment System (PPS) to control health care costs. PPS divides hospital inpatient diagnoses into 480 categories, each of which is reimbursed at a fixed rate. Medical treatments that cost more than the fixed rate are not used, as the hospital would lose money implementing the technology. Since HCFA is the largest third-party payer of health care in the United States, this reform has greatly affected the entire medical community.

In order to evade the PPS controls, many hospitals are moving operative

TABLE 3-2 Judgments of Effectiveness of Medical Applications of Lasers

Procedure	Established Clinical Experience	Randomized Controlled Trial	Probably Cost Effective	Proven Cost Effective
Dermatology				
Port-wine stain	x			
Tattoos	x			
Telangiectasia	x			
Warts	x			
Ophthalmology				
Diabetic retinopathy		x	x	x
Retinal detachment	x			
Retinal vein occlusion		x	x	
Trabeculoplasty for glaucoma		x	x	
Senile macular degeneration		x	x	
Posterior capsulotomy		x	x	
Otolaryngology				
Respiratory papillomatosis	x		x	
Pharyngeal pouch	x		x	
Tongue resections	x		x	
Pulmonology				
Palliation of advanced lung cancer	x		x	
Gastroenterology				
Hemostasis of gastric ulcer			x	
Hemostasis of intestinal vascular malformation	x			
Cancer palliation of esophagus	x		x	
Cancer palliation of colon	x		x	
Sessile villous adenomas	x			
Hemorrhoids	x		x	
Urology				
Bladder cancer	x		x	
Penile carcinoma	x		x	
Condyloma	x		x	
Laser lithotripsy	x		x	
Gynecology				
Cervical intra-epithelial neoplasia excision	x		x	
Fallopian tube reconstruction	x			
Endometriosis	x			
Condyloma	x			

SOURCE: Banta et al., 1992.

procedures to the outpatient setting, which is still reimbursed on a fee-for-service basis. The resultant trend is "minimally invasive surgery" (MIS), which includes endoscopic procedures, minor operations, and many emergency room treatments. MIS is usually cost-effective, safer, and more convenient for patients, further encouraging its development. The laser may be an important tool in this trend because its surgical effects can be very precise, minimizing damage to tissue, and because lasers can be transmitted via fiber optics with endoscopic devices. The lower costs associated with several laser procedures may lead to their adoption in the inpatient setting as well. A three-year study at Cooper Hospital/University Medical Center in Camden, New Jersey, found that lasers reduced the direct cost for gastrointestinal (GI) applications by $3,500 per patient. GI operating room expenses were reduced by 40 percent, and the average length of a hospital stay dropped from 17.7 days to 14. Similar results were found in a study of neuro-surgical, gynecological, and outpatient applications (Cerne, 1988). Still, many doctors are reluctant to use lasers; as noted about the carbon dioxide laser, "successful commercialization . . . requires the device to overcome several major hurdles, including user resistance to high system prices as well as a reluctance by physicians to replace traditional scalpels with tools requiring extensive training" (see Akerley, 1985).

Despite institutional hurdles, the medical sector is one of the fastest growing segments of the laser industry (see Table 3-3). Collaboration between laser manufacturers and clinicians has boosted medical research and equipment sales,

TABLE 3-3 Laser Sales (in million dollars)

	1985	1987	1988	1989	1990	1991	Percent Change, 1985–1991
Material processing	127.0	128.6	146.7	173.9	256.4	337.6	166
Medicine	83.7	81.0	102.8	200.2	209.5	233.8	179
R&D	104.1	123.4	141.7	216.5	218.4	190.0	83
Printing	34.2	35.8	46.5	53.2	50.8	40.0	17
Platemaking/color separation	14.2	15.4	10.9	11.4	14.1	8.4	–41
Communications	44.0	60.0	70.1	76.4	112.1	111.2	153
Optical memories	21.4	89.0	53.5	70.9	73.8	76.9	259
Barcode scanners	4.5	11.9	18.6	29.0	30.7	26.3	484
Alignment, control	2.0	0.9	5.9	7.1	7.0	10.9	445
Test and measurement	21.0	20.0	28.7	35.6	39.9	34.3	63
Entertainment	3.5	5.2	8.0	8.4	12.0	9.7	177
TOTAL	459.6	570	633.5	882.6	1,024.7	1,079.1	135

SOURCE: *Laser Focus/Electro-Optics*, 1986, 1988–1992.

and several journals have been established for this industry.[15] Such interdisciplinary collaboration between firms and academic medical doctors was essential to the success of ophthalmological lasers. No single vendor dominates the medical laser market (with the exception of argon-laser ophthalmic systems), and over 100 companies supply lasers to the medical community. In 1991, over 31,000 laser units were sold for medical and diagnostic use. Although this was less than 0.1 percent of the total number of laser units sold in the United States, the dollar value of these sales has been estimated to range from $233 million to $325 million—over 20 percent of cash sales in lasers. Ophthalmological applications dominate this purchasing, comprising $70 million of the $220 million of sales in 1988. In the United States in 1991, less than 1 percent of surgeries were performed with the laser. Advocates say that up to 50 percent could be done with laser devices (Bromberg, 1991), but recent developments have indicated that the medical market for lasers will not grow to be as large as many researchers once hoped. In 1987, C. Breck Hitz described the medical laser market as being "profitless" (Hitz, 1987) and *Laser Focus/Electro-Optics* noted that the industry had "slim profit margins" in 1989 (p. 98). The cost of bringing a new medical laser product to the consumer is still high, although the cost may decline as laser manufacturing becomes less expensive. For this reason, the laser is still considered to be in its embryonic stages in medicine.

From a laboratory in southern California, the laser has moved into nearly every medical specialty. The laser's success in ophthalmology can be traced to the research conducted by Koester and Campbell, Zaret, and Flocks, Kapany, and Zweng. These men laid the foundation for the implementation of laser techniques in medicine. They were able to do so because they had the opportunity to utilize several established methods of communication between researchers. The most important of these was the use of medical consultants by private companies. The consultancies brought physicians, physicists, and engineers together to create useful technologies for medicine. Academic medical researchers rarely have the resources or the incentive to bring a new technology to market; private companies are driven by the need to produce new devices. Also necessary in the development of the laser photocoagulator were the broad science educations obtained by Flocks, Zaret, and Campbell. Encouraging this type of education in universities could foster further collaboration between medicine and industry. Lastly, the existence of conferences and journals that cater to many scientists supported communication among and between laser developers and medical researchers.

Transferring new technological discoveries into useful medical tools is not a

---

[15]*Lasers in Surgery and Medicine* was established in the fall of 1980, *Lasers in Ophthalmology* in May 1986, *Ophthalmic Laser Therapy* in 1985, and *Lasers in Medical Science* in 1986.

deterministic process. Some dimension of serendipity is involved in the inspiration of any idea. But, as is clearly exemplified by the introduction of the laser to medicine, particular institutional structures and relationships are necessary to foster the development of medical technology. In the case of laser photocoagulation, we can thank the researchers who established relationships between private laser producers and academic medical centers for launching the development of an important tool in medicine.

ACKNOWLEDGMENTS

I am grateful to the late Milton Flocks, Narinder Kapany, Elias Snitzer, and Milton Zaret for allowing me to interview them, to Charles Koester for his correspondence, and to the Neils Bohr Library, Center for History of Physics, at the American Institute of Physics for a transcript of Joan Bromberg's interview with Elias Snitzer and a questionnaire from Charles Koester. Nathan Rosenberg and Victor Fuchs provided many useful comments. I thank the National Science Foundation for financial support.

REFERENCES

Akerley, B. H. 1985. Outlook for medical laser market strong as sales surge. *Laser Focus/Electro-Optics* 21:62–72.

Andrews, A. H., Jr. 1984. The use of the carbon dioxide laser in otolaryngology: 10 years experience. *Lasers in Surgery and Medicine* 4:305–310.

Banta, H. D., Schou, I., Vondeling, H., and de Wit, A. 1992. Economic appraisal of laser applications in health care. Report of a project. *Lasers in Medical Science* 7:9–21.

Bromberg, J. L. 1984. *Interview for the Laser History Project of Elias Snitzer.* August 6. New York: Neils Bohr Library, American Institute of Physics.

Bromberg, J. L. 1991. *The Laser in America, 1950–1970.* Cambridge, Mass.: The MIT Press.

Campbell, C. J., Koester, C., Curtice, V., Noyori, K., and Rittler, M. C. 1965. Clinical studies in laser photocoagulation. *Archives of Ophthalmology* 74:57–65.

Campbell, C. J., Noyori, K., Rittler, M. C., and Koester, C. 1963a. Intraocular temperature changes produced by laser coagulation. *Acta Ophthalmologica* 76(suppl.):22–31.

Campbell, C. J., Rittler, M. C., and Koester, C. J. 1963b. The optical maser as a retinal coagulator: An evaluation. *Transactions: American Academy of Ophthalmology and Otolaryngology* 67:58–67.

Cerne, F. 1988. Can lasers cut hospital costs? *Hospitals* 62:63.

Choy, D. S. J. 1988. History of lasers in medicine. *Thoracic and CV Surgeon* 36(suppl.2):114–117.

Cunningham, R. 1986. Applications pioneer interview: Narinder Kapany. *Lasers and Applications* 5(7):65–68.

Dunnington, J. H., Regan, E. F., and L'Esperance, F. A. 1963. Progress in Ophthalmic surgery, part 2. *New England Journal of Medicine* 269:417–413.

Foote, S. B. 1992. *Managing the Medical Arms Race: Public Policy and Medical Device Innovation.* Berkeley, Calif.: University of California Press.

Forrester, J. S. 1988. Laser angioplasty: Now and in the future. *Circulation* 78:777–779.

Goldman, L., Blaney, D., Kindel, D., and Franke, E. K. 1963a. Effect of the laser beam on the skin. *Journal of Investigative Dermatology* 40:121–122.

Goldman, L., Blaney, D. Kindel, D. J., Jr., et al. 1963b. Pathology of the effect of the laser beam on the skin. *Nature* 197:912–914.

Hall, L. T. 1990. Cardiovascular lasers: A look into the future. *American Journal of Nursing* 90(July):27–30.

Halliday, D., and Resnick, R. 1978. *Physics: Part 2.* New York: John Wiley and Sons.

Halter, P. 1985. The medical laser market waits for R & D to deliver. *Lasers and Applications* 4(October):55–57.

Ham, W. T., Jr., Williams, R. C., Geeraets, W. J., Ruffin, R. S., and Mueller, H. A. 1963. Optical masers (lasers). *Acta Ophthalmologica* 76(suppl.):60–78.

Hecht, J. 1986. Applications pioneer interview: Francis L'Esperance. *Lasers and Applications* 5(5):79–83.

Hecht, J. 1992. *Laser Pioneers.* Boston, Mass.: Academic Press, Inc.

Hitz, C. B. 1987. Medical lasers: A paradox of profitless prosperity. *Laser Focus/ Electro-Optics* 23:76–79.

Kapany, N. S., Peppers, N. A., Zweng, H. C., and Flocks, M. 1963. Retinal photocoagulation by lasers. *Nature* 199:146–149.

Kessler, D. A., Pape, S., and Sundwall, D. N. 1987. The federal regulation of medical devices. *New England Journal of Medicine* 317:357–365.

Koester, C. J., Snitzer, E., Campbell, C. J., and Rittler, M. C. 1962. Experimental laser retina photocoagulation. *Journal of the Optical Society of America* 52:607.

Laser Focus. 1965, 1967. Volumes 1, 3.

Laser Focus/Electro-Optics. 1986, 1988-1992. Volumes 22, 24–28.

L'Esperance, F. A., Jr. 1968. An ophthalmic argon laser photocoagulation system. *Transactions of the American Ophthalmological Society* 66:827–904.

L'Esperance, F. A. 1973. Argon laser photocoagulation of diabetic retinal neovascularization (a five year appraisal). *Transactions: American Academy of Ophthalmology and Otolaryngology* 77:OP6–OP24.

L'Esperance, F. A., Labuda, E. F., and Johnson, A. M. 1969. Photocoagulation delivery systems for continuous-wave lasers. *British Journal of Ophthalmology* 53:310–322.

Little, Arthur D. Decision Resources, Inc. 1989. *New Medical Laser Applications— Industry Report.* No. 948451. March 22.

Maiman, T. H. 1960. Stimulated optical radiation in ruby. *Nature* 187:493.

Meyer-Schwickerath, G. 1967. The history and development of photocoagulation. *American Journal of Ophthalmology* 63:1812–1814.

Meyer-Schwickerath, G. 1973. 25 years of photocoagulation. *Transactions: American Academy of Ophthalmology and Otolaryngology* 77:OP3–OP5.

New York Times. December 22, 1961. Light beam used in eye operation.

The Otolaryngologic Clinics of North America. 1990. Volume 23.

Proceedings of the IEEE. 1963. 57:1847–1852.

Ratz, J. L., ed. 1986. *Lasers in Cutaneous Medicine and Surgery.* Chicago: Year Book Medical Publishers, Inc.

Sanborn, T. A. 1988. Laser angioplasty: What has been learned from experimental studies and clinical trials? *Circulation* 78:769–774.

Schawlow, A. L. 1961. Optical masers. *Scientific American* 204(June):52.

Schawlow, A. L., and Townes, C. H. 1958. Infrared and optical masers. *Physics Review* 112:1940.

Sliney, D. H., and Wolbarsht, M. L. 1989. Future applications of lasers in surgery and medicine: A review. *Journal of the Royal Society of Medicine* 82:293–296.

Solon, L. R., Aronson, R., and Gould, G. 1961. Physiological implications of laser beams. *Science* 134:1506–1508.

Townes, C. 1962. Optical masers and their possible applications to biology. *Biophysics Journal* 2:325.

Trokel, S. L. 1990. Development of the excimer laser in ophthalmology. *Refractive and Corneal Surgery* 6:357–362.

Wall Street Journal. December 22, 1961. Intense beam of light from laser used successfully to treat tumor in human eye.

White, G. H. 1988. Angioscopy and lasers in CV surgery. *Australian and New Zealand Journal of Surgery* 58:271–274.

Wolbarsht, M. L., ed. 1971. *Laser Applications in Medicine and Biology.* New York: Plenum Press.

Zaret, M. M., Breinin, G. M., Schmidt, et al. 1961. Ocular lesions produced by an optical maser. *Science* 134:1525–1526.

Zaret, M. M., Ripps, H., Siegel, I. M., and Breinin, G. M. 1962. Biomedical experimentation with optical masers. *Journal of the Optical Society of America* 52:607.

Zaret, M. M., Ripps, H., Siegel, I. M., and Breinin, G. M. 1963. Laser photocoagulation of the eye. *Archives of Ophthalmology* 69:97–104.

Zweng, H. C., and Flocks, M. 1965. Clinical experiences with laser photocoagulation. *Federation Proceedings* 24:S65–S70.

Zweng, H. C., Flocks, M., and Kapany, N. S. 1964. Experimental laser photocoagulation. *American Journal of Ophthalmology* 58:353–362.

Zweng, H. C., Little, H. L., and Peabody, R. R. 1969. *Laser Photocoagulation and Retinal Angiography.* Saint Louis, Mo.: C. V. Mosby Company.

TECHNICAL APPENDIX

Until 1900, the study of light was limited to examining its behavior. Scientists had identified light sources but they did not know how light was generated. Light is commonly radiated from heated solids and gases through which an electric current is passing. Another light source is the cavity radiator, constructed of blocks of tungsten, tantalum, or molybdenum. When the blocks are heated uniformly to a high temperature, they will emit light. Max Planck (1858–1947) studied cavity radiators and from his observations defined a relation between the "radiancy" of a frequency of light, temperature, and frequency.

Planck wanted to devise a theory that would explain his formula after it was published in 1900. He believed the atoms that comprised the walls of his cavity radiator behaved like electromagnetic oscillators which emitted and absorbed electromagnetic energy. This idea led to the theory that electromagnetic oscillators (atoms) emit and absorb energy in discrete quantities. The emission and absorption of these quantities is characterized by the oscillator moving from one quantized state to another (see Halliday and Resnick, 1978).

When an electron of an atom moves from a higher quantum level (of energy, measured discretely) to a lower quantum level, a photon of energy, viewed as electromagnetic radiation, is spontaneously emitted (see Figure 3-A1). Similarly, a photon of energy can be absorbed by an electron, moving the electron to a higher quantum state. In Albert Einstein's 1916 proof of Planck's law, Einstein suggested that a photon emission might be stimulated. This idea was essentially ignored until Charles Townes proposed the maser, which was a feedback oscillator from which microwaves were emitted.

By bombarding deuterated ammonia with energy, Townes forced many of the electrons of the ND_3 atoms into higher quantum states than they normally exhibit. These atoms were enclosed in a resonator which sustained the frequency of electromagnetic emissions. The stimulated emissions were reflected back to the atoms, maintaining the high quantum states. At high levels of radiation, the device broke into self-oscillation, producing millimeter-waves continuously.

The laser is constructed in the same way as the maser described above, but with a material whose emissions produce visible light. The difficulties of creating the laser were finding an appropriate material and building a resonant chamber that would maintain the energy level of the material. Because the maser principle can be applied to many solids and gases, a wide variety of lasers exists. Each laser material produces a different wavelength of electromagnetic emission; thus, many "colors" of light can be produced with lasers (see Figure 3-A2).

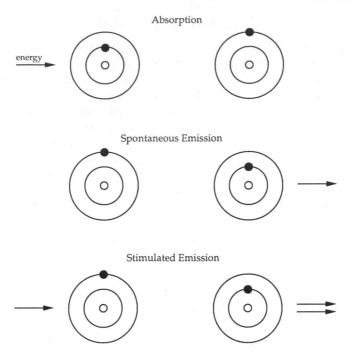

FIGURE 3-A1 Molecular absorption and emission processes.

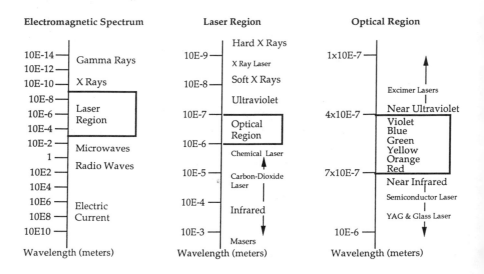

FIGURE 3-A2 "Colors" of light produced by lasers with different wavelengths.

4

From the Scalpel to the Scope: Endoscopic Innovations in Gastroenterology, Gynecology, and Surgery

ANNETINE C. GELIJNS AND NATHAN ROSENBERG

Minimally invasive therapy is an extremely dynamic area of innovation, as illustrated by the establishment of new professional journals[1] and societies, the growing number of publications in established journals as well as the lay press, and the rapid entry of medical device firms into the market. Generally, the term *innovation*—newness in its most literal sense—conveys an image of step-by-step reduction to practice of a major new scientific or engineering observation, which then generates a breakthrough technology. As the history of minimally invasive therapy shows us, however, the nature of the innovation process is much more incremental than this image suggests and, moreover, often involves the fusion of a wide range of existing technological capabilities (Kodama, 1992). Indeed, we regard as a key feature of medical innovation, and perhaps even *the* key feature, the manner in which disciplinary and organizational boundaries are crossed.

The central technological component in minimally invasive therapy is the endoscope: a slender rigid or flexible tube through which images can be transmitted, either to the eyepiece or, nowadays mostly, onto a videoscreen. A variety of accessory technologies, such as miniaturized forceps, electrocautery devices, and lasers, can then be moved through the operative channel of the endoscope, or through an alternative instrument inserted in the human body, to undertake the necessary therapeutic interventions.

---

[1] A sample of new journals includes the *Journal of Laparoscopic Surgery* (begun in 1990), *The Journal of Laparoendoscopic Surgery* (1991), *Surgical Laparoscopy & Endoscopy* (1991), *The Journal of Lithotripsy & Stone Disease* (1989), and *The Journal of Interventional Cardiology*.

In the environment of resource and cost constraint in health services that emerged during the 1980s, an uncommon consensus among patients, physicians, providers, and payers evolved regarding the rapid acceptance of this area of medical intervention, an acceptance that, in turn, has been stimulating further innovation. Minimally invasive therapy may obviate the need for major open-surgery procedures. In terms of health outcomes, it appears to offer the following advantages: elimination of the need for general anesthesia, the absence of the sequelae of open surgery procedures, minute scars, short hospital stays or outpatient treatment, and a much more rapid return to normal activity. Clearly, reductions in length of hospitalization and the ability to return to work much sooner can be regarded as attractive economic features as well. Although the current very rapid rate of diffusion and the often inadequate levels of training of clinicians in these new procedures are increasing complication rates and raising some reservations about this revolution in surgical care, minimally invasive therapy *per se* appears to promise important medical and economic benefits. Yet the history of minimally invasive therapy is a long one, and—as we shall see—these benefits were not always as obvious or important as they are nowadays.

The therapeutic use of endoscopes was preceded by their diagnostic use. In fact, since the Middle Ages, physicians had had the idea that a tube containing lenses and mirrors could be used to look into the natural orifices of the human body to obtain diagnostic information (Filipi et al., 1991). Despite these concepts and intense human curiosity, the possibility of examining the internal workings of a living body long defied human ingenuity. Natural orifices that might constitute points of entry are few. Lens systems were still unsophisticated and the only source of illumination was provided by candles or a platinum wire heated to brilliance by an electric current.[2] Even with an appropriate light source, a rigid instrument could provide little or only limited opportunity for informative inspection of certain organs, such as the digestive tract. The development of a flexible endoscope was especially beset by difficulties. Plastics were not available in the nineteenth century, and although the vulcanization of rubber, which offered a material that was strong as well as flexible, was accomplished by 1839, the major obstacle remained: finding ways to make glass lens systems flexible. Nevertheless, important advances were made in the closing decades of the nineteenth century: a critical step was Edison's discovery of the incandescent light bulb, which in miniaturized form could be mounted to the distal tip of the endoscope, and Nitze's introduction of a dramatically improved lens system. As

---

[2]In view of the primitive nature of lighting technology before the discovery of the incandescent source, the disapproval of the authorities toward attempts at visualization may not have been entirely inappropriate. As Gaskin et al. (1991) observed: "The first attempt at endoscopy was by Bozzini in 1805. He was censored by the medical faculty of Vienna for being too inquisitive in attempting to observe the interior of the urethra in a living patient with a simple tube and candlelight" (p. 1086).

a result, cystoscopy—which involved inserting a rigid endoscope into the ure-thra—became a fairly well-established procedure at this time. Around the turn of the century, efforts to develop and manufacture these endoscopes were concen-trated in Germany, a concentration that was presumably closely linked to Ger-man technical skills in the design and manufacture of instrumentation generally, and perhaps optical instruments in particular.

We should not underestimate, however, the immense gap between the per-formance of these first devices and the performance characteristics needed for more widespread adoption. For example, the lamp at the tip of the endoscope could cause serious burns, vision often was restricted, the quality of images was poor, and obtaining some form of permanent documentation of the images was highly problematic, at best. The more widespread application of endoscopic procedures required major improvements in lighting, optics, and photographic capabilities. This meant that the evolution of endoscopic techniques was essen-tially *interdisciplinary* and interinstitutional in nature; that is, it required the medical profession to create alliances with scientists and engineers with expertise in optics, electronics, and—more recently—optoelectronics. These interactions between clinicians, often in academic medical centers, and technologists, often in industrial firms, are important for the development of first-generation devices. Yet in medicine, where research and development (R&D) and adoption are closely linked, the rate and direction of the subsequent improvement process is also likely to be influenced by the experience of the early users[3] and by the effectiveness with which this information is fed back to the device manufactur-ers. Given these characteristics, our emphasis in this chapter will be on the following question: What can the history of endoscopy tell us about the circum-stances surrounding, and more specifically the barriers to, innovation that re-quires the crossing of disciplinary as well as institutional boundaries?

Before turning to the task at hand, one final point deserves mentioning. This chapter takes a historical approach in that it covers roughly half a century of innovation in endoscopy. Clearly, during this time period the economic, social, and regulatory environment within which R&D efforts have taken place under-went considerable change. Consider, for example, the economic environment. Since World War II the incentive signals from the U.S. health care financing system to the R&D sector have been to enhance quality of care regardless of costs; it is only over the past decade—with the introduction of the prospective payment system for Medicare and all kinds of managed care initiatives—that

---

[3]In medicine, the term *user* requires some clarification. Although one could argue that patients are the ultimate beneficiaries and users of technologies, patients for a variety of reasons traditionally have delegated decisions about the kinds and levels of technological intervention they need to their physi-cians. As a result, physicians have been considered the principal users insofar as the generators of new technologies are concerned.

these signals have been changing toward more emphasis on containing costs. Whereas we explore how some of these changes in the broader environment have influenced and shaped the conditions surrounding medical R&D in the past, the current changes in the incentive environments remains an important topic for further exploration.

FIBER OPTICS AND GASTROINTESTINAL ENDOSCOPY

Beginning in the 1920s, the field of gastrointestinal endoscopy in Europe and the United States was dominated by a single individual, Rudolf Schindler. Schindler, a German doctor born in Berlin in 1888, undertook hundreds of examinations with rigid gastroscopes and published his findings in a major work, *Lehrbuch und Atlas der Gastroskopie*, in 1923. He subsequently introduced a semiflexible gastroscope in 1932. His work over the next 30 years pushed the subject to what were probably the ultimate limits attainable, given the tools and materials that were available before the 1960s. The so-called Wolf-Schindler semiflexible gastroscope was "an acceptably safe, workable instrument capable of conveying informative images of the stomach's interior to the eye of the examining physician" (Haubrich, 1987, p. 6).

It is clear that Schindler relied heavily upon the skills and earlier industrial experience of George Wolf, a Berlin instrument maker. Interestingly enough, Wolf had previously devised a prototype optical instrument to be used in inspecting the condensing tubes in steam engines. His acquired skills in conveying light rays along a flexible arc were central to the achievement of the gastroscope. However, it was Schindler's basic ideas that eventually prevailed. Wolf had at first "proposed and constructed an optical gastroscope that was flexible throughout its length, but Schindler had the better idea of combining a rigid proximal half with a flexible distal half, thus producing a more wieldy instrument that conveyed a brighter, clearer image. The result was the famous Wolf-Schindler semiflexible gastroscope" (Haubrich, 1987, p. 6).[4]

Schindler, who was half Jewish, managed to escape Nazi Germany in 1934 and continued his practice and teaching of endoscopy in Chicago and, eventually, Los Angeles. His textbook, *Gastroscopy*, published in 1937 and in revised editions in 1950 and 1966, was "the gospel of gastroscopy for a generation of clinicians" (Haubrich, p. 6). While in Chicago, Schindler continued to be absorbed in ways of improving both the design and the construction of the gastroscope. As he had done with Wolf in Berlin, he formed a close connection with William J. Cameron. Cameron's firm, the Cameron Surgical Company, "became the world's largest supplier of illuminated instruments" (Haubrich, p. 7). Schindler

---

[4]Patients may have opted for some modifier other than "semiflexible."

worked especially closely with Louis Streifeneder, a talented instrument maker from Cameron's firm, who later formed his own company (the Eder Instrument Company) for producing high-quality laparoscopes. During World War II, with German instruments no longer available, Cameron's company introduced the Cameron Omniangle Gastroscope, a modification of the Wolf-Schindler gastroscope, which became a widely used standard instrument in the United States.

It seems clear that, both in Germany and the United States, Schindler was responsible for numerous initiatives in the improved design of the gastroscope, in addition to his pioneering role in introducing it as a tool for extracting information from the patient's gastrointestinal (GI) tract. But the difficulties and limitations in gastroscopy before the advent of fiber optics are hard to exaggerate. It remained an unusual diagnostic procedure. At best, it afforded the examiner fleeting and partial visual impressions of only portions of the stomach as the gastroscopist attempted to manipulate a semiflexible instrument, with an incandescent light bulb at its distal tip, inside the gut of a (presumably) very uncomfortable and apprehensive patient.

The innovation that was responsible for the transformation in endoscopy that began in the 1950s was the emergence of fiber optics. In principle, fiber optics allowed the design of flexible endoscopes, which offered the technical possibility of providing visual inspection of internal organs that were not readily accessible with rigid instruments or that were accessible to only a limited degree with the use of Schindler-type semiflexible endoscopes, for example, the duodenal bulb. The earliest applications of this new capability were on the GI tract, where flexibility was essential. But, as we will see, flexible endoscopy later had applications elsewhere where flexibility was also a critical feature.

The Fiber-Optic Era

Scientific research on the properties of light that are relevant to fiber-optic endoscopy has a long history. Fiber optics make it possible to transmit both light and images along a curved path through the use of bundles of long thin fibers of optical glass. The basic science underlying light transmission had been first expounded by the great Dutch scientist Christiaan Huygens in the seventeenth century. His formulation of the wave theory of light provided an explanation of refraction (bending) and reflection (Salmon, 1974). In 1870, at the Royal Society, John Tyndall demonstrated experimentally how light could be conducted along a curved path, the curved path in this case being a stream of water. Further experimentation was conducted in the 1920s and 1930s, and a patent on a technique for transmitting light through flexible quartz or glass fiber bundles had been taken out by Logie Baird in England in 1928. But these experiments led to no immediate useful applications.

Fiber-optic endoscopy had its origins in the early 1950s, when research was begun on the possibility of transmitting images along an aligned bundle of flexible glass fibers. The findings of A. C. S. van Heel in Holland and H. H. Hopkins and his student, N. S. Kapany, in the department of physics at the Imperial College in London were simultaneously reported in *Nature* (Hopkins and Kapany, 1954; van Heel, 1954). These papers laid down the principles of coherent image transmission by means of fiber optics. Van Heel presented the concept of the coated glass fiber, although he discussed only the possibility of plastic coatings, which later turned out to be unsatisfactory. Both papers described a way of conveying optical images along a glass fiber—a concept that had an earlier history—but Hopkins and Kapany also elucidated the basic principles of fiber alignment. In these 1954 papers the authors made the linkage between their research and medicine; Hopkins and Kapany, for instance, observed that "[a]n obvious use of the unit is to replace the train of lenses employed in conventional endoscopes" (Hopkins and Kapany, 1954). It is important to observe that the work of van Heel and of Hopkins and Kapany was possible at this time because of major recent improvements in the manufacture of glass that had the effect of reducing the loss of light in transmission.

If there is a single critical event in the early development of fiber-optic endoscopy, it was the reading of the *Nature* articles of Hopkins and Kapany and of van Heel by Basil Hirschowitz. Hirschowitz, a young South African gastroenterologist, went to the University of Michigan in 1953 on an American Cancer Society fellowship. Hirschowitz received some training in endoscopy as a medical student at the University of Witwatersrand and later at the Central Middlesex Hospital in London. He was very much aware of the limitations of the Schindler semiflexible gastroscope for upper GI endoscopy: "Half of the instrument could be flexed for introduction into the oesophagus, but once in the stomach, it had to be straight to accommodate the 50 or more lenses spaced along the shaft. Gastroscopy with the Schindler instrument required good training, a good assistant, and a patient with a compliant anatomy approaching that of a sword swallower" (Hirschowitz, 1989, pp. 247–250).

According to Hirschowitz, from the time of his arrival at the University of Michigan Hospital in 1953 "we had become disenchanted with conventional upper GI rigid and semi-rigid endoscopy and more often than not the prevailing attitude in gastroenterology was to avoid rather than encourage its use" (Hirschowitz, 1989, p. 247). Discussions with C. Wilbur Peters, an optical physicist at the University of Michigan, convinced him of the feasibility of developing a fiber-optic instrument for visualizing the upper GI tract. In the summer of 1954, Hirschowitz visited Hopkins and Kapany in London where he examined their glass fiber bundle. The glass was inappropriate. It was commercially available glass of a kind used for glass cloth. It did indeed transmit an image, but was far from the stage of a practical instrument: "Light transmission was inadequate to produce the requisite one meter length for an endoscopy, the colour of the light transmitted was green, and the image was not sharp" (Hirschowitz,

1989, p. 248). Nevertheless, Hirschowitz was persuaded that a workable instrument was attainable.

Back at the University of Michigan, a young sophomore student by the name of Larry Curtiss was made a part of the team. It is worth observing at this point that Hirschowitz thought of the University of Michigan as a place where interdisciplinary communication and research was relatively easy. He recalled, "Ann Arbor was an exciting place to work, with bright, eager young men in various medical and non-medical disciplines. Interdisciplinary attitudes were strong at Michigan. For example, a group of about 10 of us used to meet one evening a week to discuss our research and to brainstorm over a can or two of beer" (Hirschowitz, 1979, pp. 864–869).

Peters, Curtiss, and Hirschowitz confronted numerous difficulties. The fiber glass available at that time was inadequate and there was no commercially available apparatus for forming the fiber bundles. Fortunately, through Hirschowitz's connection with someone at the Corning Corporation in Midland, Michigan, they were given access to a supply of optical glass rods. Peters, Curtiss, and Hirschowitz then put together, from miscellaneous materials in the physics department basement, an apparatus for making fiber.

A number of problems remained to be solved, including the proper orientation and protection of the fibers and the polishing of the ends to attain flat optical entry and exit surfaces. More serious difficulties centered on "cross talk" (i.e., when fibers come into contact light jumps from one fiber to another, leading to loss in image transmission). A crucial problem, then, was to develop a technique for insulating the fibers to eliminate cross talk.

Eventually, by December 1956, Curtiss, the undergraduate, found a solution to the insulation problem. It was glass-coated glass fiber. Essentially, what he did was "to melt a rod of optical glass inside a tube of lower refractive index glass and pull the two together into a composite fiber" (Hirschowitz, 1979, p. 866). This provided a solution to the problems of insulation and excessive light loss. According to Hirschowitz, "That invention is the single most important optical advance in endoscopy. From then on it was purely a matter of applying and developing the process—we were home free" (Hirschowitz, 1979, p. 866).

Hirschowitz tested the first operating gastroscope upon himself in February 1957: "I looked at this rather thick, forbidding but flexible rod, took the instrument and my courage in both hands, and swallowed it over the protests of my unanesthetized pharynx and my vomiting center" (Hirschowitz, 1979, p. 866). A few days later he used it to examine a patient suffering from a duodenal ulcer.

Significantly, in view of the great impact it was to have in just a few years, the fiberscope generated little interest at first, even at the meeting of the American Gastroscopic Society in Colorado Springs in May 1957. (Schindler was in attendance. Kapany, who was also at the meeting, reported that the firm Bausch and Lomb, with whom he was working, would soon introduce its own fiberscope. They never did so.) Nor was there any initial enthusiasm among instrument manufacturers, either in the United States or England. Eventually American Cystoscope Makers, Inc. (ACMI), which had tried unsuccessfully to make usable fiber-optic bundles, undertook to manufacture fiberscopes, under license, but only if Curtiss, Peters, and Hirschowitz would agree to act as consultants. The agreement called for Curtiss and Peters "to get the glass-fiber making off the ground with ACMI engineering staff" (Hirschowitz, 1979, p. 867). It should be particularly noted, then, that the academic/medical trio at the University of Michigan not only solved a critical technological problem with respect to the new device— the cladding of the glass fiber—but they were also instrumental in teaching the industrial firm how to solve some complicated manufacturing problems—the making of the fiber-optic bundles. This is a drastic departure from what might be regarded as the "normal" division of labor between academics and instrument manufacturers.

The initial skepticism that greeted Hirschowitz's prototype fiberscope was hardly unusual. As suggested earlier, innovations commonly enter the world with poor performance characteristics and they often require years of attention and patient development work before they assert their technical superiority. This was graciously yet, at the same time, revealingly acknowledged, in the case of the fiberscope, by William Haubrich, himself an eminent authority on endoscopy:

> I recall having been shown this prototype instrument on a visit to Hirschowitz's laboratory. It was rigged so as to convey the visage of Abraham Lincoln that adorned a 5 cent stamp. Peering into the fiberscope, I could not deny recognizing Lincoln, but the quality of the image reminded me of a picture I had seen of prototype television images displayed in the 1920s. Vivid it was not. Comparing this with the image then obtained by the lens-and-prism gastroscope, I confess I saw little future in fiberoptic endoscopy. A remarkable accomplishment, I thought, but little will come of it. Now, along with thousands of other endoscopists the world over, I rejoice in my lack of prescience (Haubrich, 1987, p. 13).

The instrument went through a succession of improvements in four or five months until the so-called Mark V, the ACMI 4990 Hirschowitz fiberscope ("the model T of fiber-optic endoscopy") was introduced. The results of its early use were reported in *Lancet* in May 1961, accompanied by color photographs. Such photographs were extremely important for purposes of documentation.[5]

---

[5]In the *Lancet* article Hirschowitz stated: "The application of fibre optics to the examination of the upper gastro-intestinal tract has opened new dimensions in diagnostic endoscopy. Areas not previously accessible are now readily displayed—the pyloric canal, the duodenal bulb, and both afferent and efferent loops of the jejunum through the gastroenterostomy stoma. These areas can not only be studied for abnormalities but also for motility for comparatively long periods. Furthermore, the complete flexibility of the fiberscope means that examination is very much easier for the patient, and introduction of the instrument requires no special skill. More important, damage to the oesophagus or stomach, particularly the oesophagus, is no longer a consideration as it was with the conventional gastroscope. Thus, many more patients can be examined easily and safely and the indications for its use should be much broader" (Hirschowitz, 1961, pp. 1074–1078).

Firms other than ACMI attempted to develop and manufacture flexible endoscopes. The American entrants, such as the Eder Instrument Company, had no success (Louis Steifeneder, founder of the company, had, as we have seen, worked with Schindler at an earlier period). American Optical Company did introduce a flexible endoscope, but a long patent infringement suit, eventually won by ACMI, developed between ACMI and American Optical (AO). Whereas ACMI had filed patents in the United States and Europe, it had not filed a patent in Japan, which is surprising in view of the fact that GI problems had long constituted a major health problem in that country. During the 1960s, AO licensed the technology to the Olympus Corporation of Japan and to Machida Instrument Company, which were already producing semirigid endoscopes.

The Japanese firms, in particular Olympus, had also developed a gastro-camera even before the introduction of the fiberscope. The ability to obtain good color photographs of the GI tract was extremely important for documentation, as well as for consultation, and for teaching purposes. Photographs and even moving pictures had long been considered and attempted, with no particular success. For many years the best visual representation of gastric anomalies had been the work of artists. The gastrocamera was developed by T. Uji, working with Olympus. Olympus introduced the gastrocamera as early as 1955, and it came into widespread use in Japan by the early 1960s. According to Haubrich (1987, p. 11), there were 10,000 gastrocameras in Japan in 1966. The gastrocamera reflected the remarkable Japanese skills in camera miniaturization, and it took pictures of extremely high quality.

The gastrocamera, however, had severe limitations. The camera was attached to the tip of the endoscope. It took pictures from a number of preset positions, and the operator could inspect the contents of the patient's stomach only after the film had been developed. Moreover, swallowing a camera, even a miniaturized one, remained a distinctly unwieldy and unpleasant experience. The gastrocamera was never widely adopted in the United States, in spite of the efforts of John Morrissey of the University of Wisconsin (Perna et al., 1965). It was overtaken by the improvements in fiber-optic technology: "[A]s the optical system of the fiberscope was rapidly improved, it soon thereafter became much easier for most endoscopists to simply attach an external 35 mm camera to the eyepiece of the gastroscope and photograph the image conveyed by the fiber bundle. . . . The gastrocamera, marvelous as it was, became obsolete" (Perna at al., 1965).

Further Refinements and New Clinical Applications

In the late 1960s fiber-optic endoscopes were refined in many ways: "Among notable improvements were those of optical clarity, in wieldiness and manipulability of the distal tip, and in provision of channels for biopsy and therapeutic maneuvers. The Japanese were especially intent on this work because of the need to precisely diagnose gastric cancer" (Haubrich, 1987, pp. 11–13). Within a short period of time fiber-optic techniques were being used "to inspect any and all cavities and potential cavities in the body" (Hirschowitz, 1979, p. 868). It is particularly appropriate, in accordance with our emphasis on the interdisciplinary aspect of this technology, that one of the early applications of this newly developed capability was a special gastroscope developed in 1962 that would allow Rolls Royce to inspect the interior of aircraft engines without having to undertake expensive and time-consuming dismantling.

After its initial successes in the upper GI tract, fiber-optic technology quickly spread to other gastroenterological uses. Employing a fiber-optic bundle with a working length of 75 centimeters (cm), the esophagoscope—an end-viewing modification of Hirschowitz's side-viewing fiberscope—became the first fiber-optic endoscope to achieve widespread use. After the working length of the fiberscope was extended to 110 cm "we had an easily insertible instrument with which the esophagus, stomach, and duodenum could be scrutinized all in the same procedure" (Haubrich, 1987, p. 13).

Fiber-optic endoscopy has been of particular value in colonoscopy, where flexibility is essential. The extremely sharp curvature of the sigmoid colon rendered it inaccessible to examination with a rigid, lens-and-prism endoscope. Before fiber optics, proctosigmoidoscopes could inspect only 25–30 cm of the proctosigmoid. Fiberoptic colonoscopy originated in the 1960s at the academic medical center of the University of Michigan, where Hirschowitz had done his earlier work. It was pioneered by Bergein Overholt. Overholt reported the results of his first examinations at the 1967 meeting of the American Society for Gastrointestinal Endoscopy. An important feature of the application of endoscopy to the examination of the colon is that it led very quickly to a new therapeutic procedure of great value: polypectomy. Since polyps, especially multiple polyps, sometimes turn malignant, the opportunity to diagnose and to maintain regular surveillance is extremely valuable.

Overholt reports that the U.S. Public Health Service awarded a grant to Optics Technology, Inc., of California for the development of a flexible sigmoidoscope (the president of this company was N. S. Kapany, who had moved from London to the United States, eventually to California). This early attempt at design and development was unsuccessful: "[I]t became apparent that more information on the anatomy of the colon was needed for engineers to develop instrument prototypes" (Overholt, 1981, p. 2). Important assistance in securing this information was provided by Dow-Corning Aid to Medical Research. As Overholt observes: "Although many companies became interested in this new field, it was the Illinois Institute of Technology Research Institute and the Eder Instrument Company that developed the first successful prototypes of the flexible fibreoptic sigmoidoscope. After somewhat difficult trials in animals, clinical experimentation began" (Overholt, 1981, p. 3).

Parallel development work was being conducted in Japan during the 1960s, with early colon fiberscope prototypes being designed by clinicians in cooperation with Machida and Olympus. Nevertheless, "the first true colonoscope" was developed by ACMI in the late 1960s. The technique of colonoscopic polypectomy was first introduced by Hiromi Shinya, working at the Beth Israel and Mt. Sinai Medical Centers in New York, in 1969. By 1982, Dr. Shinya could report that he had "performed approximately 45,000 colonoscopies and more than 10,000 polypectomies for various lesions larger than 0.5 cm in diameter" (Shinya, 1982, p. v.). Dr. Shinya "made the outstanding contribution of polypectomy using an expandable wire-loop snare inserted through a channel of the colonoscope. Shinya was able to remove polyps safely, thus avoiding the necessity of repeated barium enema observation and transabdominal colotomy for polypectomy" (Overholt, 1981, p. 5). In this way, the technology of diagnosis had also become a direct part of the technology of therapy.

Another application in which endoscopy moved from being a diagnostic to a therapeutic technology is in bile duct stones. During the early 1950s, the Richard Wolf Company had introduced a choledochoscope that could be used *during* surgery for visualizing the interior of the common duct. In subsequent years, the German optics company Karl Storz introduced an improved rigid choledochoscope and ACMI a flexible fiber-optic choledochoscope (Wildegans, 1960). Yet despite these advances, surgeons were reluctant to adopt routine use of this procedure. Initial sources of this reluctance included concern about possible increases in operating time, rates of wound infection, and other morbidity. Failure to appreciate the high incidence of retained stones and difficulties in changing a routine may also have played a role.

A major step forward in diagnosis came with the introduction of endoscopic retrograde cholangiopancreatography (ERCP) in 1970 in Japan (Oi et al., 1970). This technique involved moving an endoscope through the duodenum and then in retrograde manner into the biliary tract to view the common duct. Development and manufacturing of these endoscopes were undertaken by Olympus and Machida. Gastroenterologists in Japan and also in Germany began experimental animal work to test the endoscope as a therapeutic tool in the common bile duct. Because in the early 1970s surgical intervention in the case of recurrent or retained common duct stones carried a significantly high mortality risk, there was a clear need for a safer procedure. Risks were especially high for elderly and frail patients with comorbidities. Thus, in 1974, gastroenterologists from university clinics in Germany and Japan for the first time extended the use of ERCP from diagnosis to therapy in this patient group. This technique, a so-called endoscopic sphincterotomy, soon demonstrated considerable advantages over operation procedures for duct stones and, as practitioners acquired the necessary skills, clinical results improved (Classen and Demling, 1974; Kawai et al., 1974).

During the late 1970s, video-guided endoscopy had become reality with the introduction of add-on television cameras to the endoscope and videorecorders for the permanent storage of images. A revolutionary change, however, was embodied in a prototype colonoscope that was first introduced for clinical testing in 1983 by the firm Welch Allyn (Classen and Phillip, 1984). In this prototype the optical fiber bundle was replaced by a charge couple device (CCD), a kind of microprocessor chip, at the distal tip of the endoscope. This chip can convert the intensity and color of light into a digitalized signal that is electronically transmitted to a videoprocessor for display on the television monitor. This integrated video-endoscopy system offered the advantages of superior images and reduction in manufacturing costs, because a microprocessor chip is far less expensive to produce than an optical fiber bundle. The CCD was invented by W. S. Boyle and G. E. Smith in 1969 and—as these academicians had not filed a patent—it was available to all manufacturers. Following the patent on the CCD-colonoscope by Welch Allyn and the introduction into practice of its colonoscope and gastroscope, the Storz firm and Japanese manufacturers, such as Fujinon, Pentax, and Olympus, introduced their versions of integrated videoendoscopes. These companies quickly overtook Welch Allyn; in particular, Olympus, by taking advantage of its video technology developed in nonmedical markets, became the leading manufacturer. Moving from gastroenterology to gynecology, we can observe that the different technological requirements of these specialties affected R&D priorities and the mix of firms involved.

GYNECOLOGICAL LAPAROSCOPY:
THE CASE OF SURGICAL CONTRACEPTION

Intra-abdominal procedures used to (and still) involve considerable trauma to patients as well as lengthy periods of hospitalization. These characteristics stimulated clinicians early on to search for alternative interventions, particularly for exploratory or diagnostic surgery. Around the turn of the century internists had begun to insert a rigid endoscope (also called a laparoscope) through a small incision for visualizing the upper abdominal organs (Gunning, 1974). Kelling, for instance, reported his first laparoscopic examination of a dog in 1901. At around the same time, the Russian Ott and the Swede Jacobeus began to apply laparoscopy as a diagnostic procedure in humans. The use of laparoscopes for diagnosis of liver and gallbladder disease was particularly stimulated by the German internist Kalk, who during the 1930s made major improvements in the lens systems involved (Kalk, 1929).[6]

Developing and Establishing the Clinical Value of First-Generation
Gynecological Laparoscopes (1945–1960s)

The transfer of diagnostic laparoscopy to gynecology, however, did not oc-

---

[6]It is interesting to note that such diagnostic laparoscopy was largely replaced by the subsequent introduction of ultrasound and other imaging techniques.

cur very rapidly, mainly because there are more vital organs and blood vessels in the human pelvis than in the upper abdomen—rendering gynecological applications more risky (Semm, 1977). The first attempts to introduce laparoscopy in gynecology can be attributed to the French gynecological surgeon Palmer, who reported on his first 250 patients in 1947 (Palmer, 1947). Palmer used the laparoscope for diagnostic purposes (including biopsy of ovarian tissue) and simple operative procedures, the most common of which was female sterilization.[7] Until that date, such contraception was provided by an abdominal operation called a laparotomy. Whereas these laparotomies had become relatively safe and effective over time, they still needed to be performed under general anesthesia, left a major abdominal scar, and involved hospitalization. To circumvent these drawbacks, gynecologists developed colpotomy, which required a vaginal incision to reach the fallopian tubes (Wortman and Piotrow, 1973). This operation indeed could be carried out under spinal anesthesia, left no visible scar, and required less hospitalization, but involved a considerable level of postoperative infections.

As the above indicates, the stage was thus set for the development of an alternative that could address these disadvantages. The first step in Palmer's laparoscopic procedure was to insert a needle into the abdomen, which was then inflated with room air. This insufflation separated the abdominal wall from the abdominal organs, providing space for introduction of the laparoscope. The laparoscope was inserted through a trocar into the abdomen. After its insertion, Palmer made another incision through which he inserted a tube with the instruments needed for cutting and ligating the fallopian tubes. Clearly, applying sutures through a slender tube required a considerable amount of surgical skill. In the early 1950s, Palmer and colleagues at a few other European centers started to collaborate with two newly established endoscope manufacturers (the German optics companies Richard Wolf and Karl Storz) to develop clinically useful gynecological laparoscopes. These centers included two in Germany—Frangenheim's group in Konstanz and, somewhat later, gynecologist K. Semm's department at the University of Kiel. In the United Kingdom, P. Steptoe became one of the early proponents of gynecological laparoscopy.

At that time, their American counterparts took an alternative developmental route by focusing their efforts on culdoscopy. Culdoscopy contains elements of both laparoscopy and colpotomy in that an endoscope called a culdoscope is inserted through a vaginal incision. The procedure was first described in 1940 by the renowned professor of obstetrics and gynecology TeLinde; the gynecologist Decker contributed much to its subsequent development with the above-mentioned firm ACMI (Rioux, 1989). This procedure also involves inserting two instruments: after the culdoscope is inserted to view the tubes, a second instru-

---

[7]The first proposal to use laparoscopic contraception can be attributed to Bösch in Switzerland and Anderson in the United States in the mid-1930s (Anderson, 1937; Liskin et al., 1985).

ment is used to bring the tubes through the incision into direct view for ligation or other methods of tubal occlusion.

The adoption of both these procedures was very limited in the 1950s, mainly as a result of significant technical and clinical limitations (Semm, 1987). One important limitation was that the early endoscopes had a lamp at the tip of the endoscope, which could lead to serious burns when they were introduced into body cavities. Operative vision was often restricted, the quality of the image poor, and it was highly difficult to obtain photographs. Moreover, laparoscopy carried additional risks because it required the creation of a pneumoperitoneum without a reliable way to monitor gas flow and pressure. In addition, insufflation of atmospheric air introduced the risk of air emboli and, as endotracheal inhalation anesthesia had not yet been developed, anesthesia was often risky.

The more widespread acceptance of these procedures in gynecological practice depended on advances in three major technical areas: lighting and optics, insufflation, and photography. In addition, their therapeutic use required the development of instruments for grasping, cutting, ligation, and coagulation. The introduction of fiber optics provided a major improvement in illumination. In 1952, Fourestier, Gladu, and Vulmière provided the first description of a fiber-optic bronchoscope that transmitted intense but cool light along a quartz-silicon rod from the proximal to the distal end of the device. They concluded their paper with the observation that "nous sommes convaincus que les résultats que nous avons obtenus dans l'exploration endobronchique se retrouveront dans toutes les autres endoscopies médicales" (Fourestier et al., 1952). A gynecological version of this fiber-optic endoscope was developed by Palmer in conjunction with the Wolf firm, and Storz introduced its "cold-light" endoscope a few years later in 1960.

It is interesting to note that R&D priorities for gastroenterological and gynecological endoscopy started to diverge at this time. In the area of gastroenterology, the need for a flexible endoscope focused R&D efforts on fiber optics as a means of image transmission. In the area of gynecology, and other medical fields that use rigid endoscopes, the major improvement in optics was the introduction of the rod-lens system by the earlier mentioned optical physicist Hopkins, now at the University of Reading (British patent no. 954629). Lens systems in conventional endoscopes consisted of a tube of air interspaced with glass lenses, which was found to absorb rather than transmit the majority of light. The revolutionary change in the Hopkins system was that it employed a tube of glass with thin air lenses. Advantages of the new endoscope were a major increase in light transmission and a wider viewing angle, which meant that examination time could be decreased. In addition, the rod-lens system allowed one to decrease the diameter of the endoscope without diminishing the quality of the image. This miniaturization of the endoscope meant that smaller trocars could be used, which reduced injuries (Berci et al., 1973). The Hopkins endoscope was introduced by Storz in 1966. Storz also worked closely with the German gynecologist Semm, who developed an automatic insufflation device to monitor the pneumoperitoneum in the early 1960s. Another step forward in the area of insufflation was the substitution of room air by carbon dioxide (CO_2) or nitrous oxygen, which reduced air emboli (Semm, 1987).

The improved illumination provided by fiber optics and the Hopkins lens system permitted advances in the documentation of endoscopic images to occur. The need for objective records had been recognized since the late 1800s: diagnostic accuracy would be considerably improved if a physician could compare photographs of a patient at different time intervals. Such photographs could also be used for teaching and, perhaps more importantly, as a means for convincing colleagues that endoscopes were valuable clinical tools. Yet, the practical implementation of this need was beset by difficulties. Originally, a miniature flash tube had to be inserted into the body cavity together with the endoscope, and a bulky and heavy camera had to be attached to its eyepiece (Berci et al., 1973). In the mid-1950s, Storz introduced an electronic flash device that was adjacent to the eyepiece and substantially improved photographic capability. However, when taking repeated pictures the eyepiece tended to heat up; Wolf addressed this problem by using the fiber-optic cable to transmit the electronic flash to the lens. Existing endoscope manufacturers also paid much attention to miniaturization of the camera and the development of an easy means of coupling the camera to the endoscope. In addition to still photography, the potential of movie cameras was explored. Cinematography required further improvements in illumination and the development of a special lightweight movie camera. A number of prototype devices were developed, but effective scaling up for production could not be obtained.

The invention of television therefore stimulated great interest. Among its advantages were that the image did not need to be developed first but could be viewed immediately by the whole operating team. Moreover, the image could be enlarged and corrected, and viewed in a binocular fashion. Finally, the image could be recorded from the screen with a normal camera or a movie camera. The first clinical experiment was performed by the physician Soulas during a bronchoscopy procedure by using a heavy Orthicon studiocamera (Soulas, 1956). In subsequent experiments, the smaller industrial Vidicon cameras were used, but they still weighed between three and six pounds. In the late 1950s, the Australian physicians Berci and Davids started to design and develop a small prototype camera that could be easily coupled to the endoscope (Berci and Davids, 1962). Berci subsequently moved to the United States and proceeded with his work on a black and white TV camera with the engineer Jack Urban, the president of a small engineering company. They developed a prototype lightweight TV camera for use in various rigid endoscopes, which would be later manufactured by ACMI. In the 1960s, however, black and white TV cameras were not yet widely available for endoscopic uses, and color television was definitely highly experimental.

Finally, various methods of occluding the fallopian tubes were developed other than applying sutures, which required considerable skill and dexterity. In 1962, Palmer described the use of laparoscopy with unipolar electrocoagulation for tubal occulation (Palmer, 1962). An advantage was its effectiveness; a disadvantage was that burns to other organs could occur. A nonelectrical alternative was the development of clips. One of the earliest clips was the tantalum hemoclip, which was originally designed to occlude vessels during surgery.

Following the introduction of these advances, laparoscopy was embraced more widely in gynecological practice, first in Europe and then in the United States—as illustrated by the establishment of the American Association for Gynecological Laparoscopists in 1971 (Steptoe, 1967).[8] Feedback from users indicated that laparoscopy had a number of advantages over laparotomy (Liskin et al., 1985). For example, it could be performed under spinal or local anesthesia and on an outpatient or day-stay basis with reduced costs; other advantages were that it involved only minute scars, minimal discomfort, and rapid recovery to normal activity. At the same time, a number of drawbacks emerged. Laparoscopy, for example, required two punctures for the insertion of instruments, which was time-consuming and increased risks. A rare but serious side effect occurring with unipolar electrocoagulation was burns to other organs. The tantalum clips used as a nonelectrical alternative also had their problems: they did not always block the tubes completely, leading to unacceptable failure rates and the serious risk of ectopic pregnancies. Furthermore, photographic capabilities were in need of improvement.

Development of Second- and Third-Generation Procedures (1970s and 1980s)

The rapidly increasing levels of adoption of gynecological laparoscopy, both for diagnostic and sterilization purposes, increased industrial interest. In addition to the existing manufacturers Wolf, Storz, and ACMI, the U.S. Eder Instrument Company and KLI (later to become Cabot Medical) and the German Winter & IBE entered the market. These firms worked with gynecologists to address the problems encountered with first-generation laparoscopic procedures. In 1972, for example, the gynecologist Wheeless designed and perfected the operating laparoscope, which allowed a physician to view as well as obstruct the tubes with one instrument, thus preventing the need for a second puncture (Wheeless, 1972). Endoscopic firms started to manufacture both operating laparoscopes and laparoscopes for double-puncture procedures.

In addition, improvements in cinematographic and television systems were made. With better lighting owing to high-intensity halogen light sources and

---

[8]Culdoscopy, which was more widely used in the United States, was found to have more side effects than laparoscopy, and it was also more difficult to perform. Its use therefore diminished during the 1970s.

Wolf's lumina optic system, color movies became a realistic option (Berci et al., 1973). Around the mid-1970s, endoscopic manufacturers also introduced a range of black and white TV cameras. In certain areas of endoscopy, especially those where inflammatory processes are prevalent, visualization of natural color is very important. Color television was still in its infancy and plagued by problems of inadequate resolution, high cost, and the size and weight of the television system. It was only in the late 1970s to early 1980s that small and lightweight color television cameras were manufactured that could be easily coupled to the eyepiece of the endoscope and that allowed a reasonable display of the image on the television screen. With the introduction of videorecorders, these images could be stored for future reference.

These endoscope manufacturers also began to focus their R&D efforts on developing a wide range of instruments that could be moved through the operative channel of the endoscope or any other cannula being used. Close cooperation with gynecologists was especially important in this area. Storz, for example, collaborated successfully with Semm at the University of Kiel. Kurt Semm had been trained as both a gynecologist and an engineer. As this suggests, one effective way of overcoming interdisciplinary boundaries is for one single person to acquire professional competence in both disciplines. With Storz, he designed needle holders, better trocars, hook scissors, irrigation and aspiration systems, and intra- and extracorporeal knot-tying instruments, to name but a few. These instruments played a vital role in the development and further popularization of gynecological laparoscopy. Through Storz's ability to create close collaborations with Semm as well as the physicist Hopkins, this firm became the leading manufacturer in gynecological laparoscopes, holding 40 percent of the world market. At the same time, ACMI—which was diverting its energy to competing with Japanese firms in the gastroenterological area—dropped out of the gynecological field.

A different set of firms manufactured energy sources used for electrocoagulation, which also underwent considerable improvement. To eliminate the burns that occurred with unipolar coagulation, the French gynecologist Rioux developed bipolar electrocoagulation (Rioux and Cloutier, 1974). The emergence of the bipolar technique and the use of low-voltage, high-frequency generators substantially diminished side effects. Another development that originated in Semm's clinic was thermocoagulation, which destroys the tubes by heat rather than electricity (Semm, 1987). Important manufacturers included some traditional large electrosurgical companies, such as Birtcher, Cameron-Miller, and Downs. Concerns about inadvertent burns also stimulated the development of a wide variety of mechanical occlusive devices. There are two types of mechanical devices: clips and rings. Repeated modifications of the tantalum clip resulted in the design of the spring-loaded clip by the gynecologist Hulka and the bioengineer Clemens, first used in 1972 (Hulka et al., 1973). The fallope or tubal ring is the most widely used occlusive device. It was developed by Bae Yoon in 1973 at Johns Hopkins University in collaboration with KLI (Yoon and King, 1975).

The popularity of surgical contraception increased steadily during the 1970s; in 1982, for instance, it became the most commonly used contraceptive method in the United States (Liskin et al., 1985). With improvements in instrumentation and techniques, gynecologists started using laparoscopes for more complex operative procedures, such as the evaluation of treated pelvic malignancies, lysis of pelvic adhesions, treatment of infertility, and laparoscopic removal of the ovaries (Semm, 1987). With this transition came demand for more sophisticated equipment. Gynecologists, for example, wanted better tools for dissecting and coagulation, and started to adopt lasers during the early 1980s. These more complex procedures also required that the other members of the team be able to observe the operation and provide useful assistance. At the same time, demand for video-guided endoscopy came from another specialty: orthopedic surgeons started to perform arthroscopy for diagnosis and treatment of disease of the joints in the late 1970s.

Existing leading manufacturers of rigid endoscopes, such as Storz and Wolf, focused on meeting this demand, but these new requirements opened opportunities for new firms to enter the laparoscopy/arthroscopy arena. Stryker, a firm with a history in medical video imaging, entered the endoscopy field and became very strong in the manufacturing of arthroscopes. The rapid growth in gynecological and other applications of rigid endoscopes also stimulated Japanese firms that had been prominent innovators in the development of flexible fiber-optic endoscopes, such as Olympus, Machida, and Fujinon, to extend their R&D efforts to rigid endoscopes (e.g., in the early 1980s, Olympus bought the firm Winter & IBE). Given the strengths of these new firms in medical video applications (using CCD endoscopes), these firms were well-positioned to make the transition to surgical laparoscopy.

THE SURGEON AND ENDOSCOPY:
LAPAROSCOPIC CHOLECYSTECTOMY

Despite the increasingly extensive use of endoscopes and laparoscopes by gastroenterologists and gynecologists, the general surgeon did not adopt these tools until the late 1980s. What were the reasons for this time lag? In part they were of a technical nature: as mentioned, it was difficult to undertake more complex surgical procedures before the introduction of video endoscopy. In 1985, for example, Filipi and colleagues ended their animal experiments with laparoscopic cholecystectomy because of the absence of video systems (Filipi et al., 1991). Yet another—and probably more important—reason was that the development and adoption of surgical endoscopy was shaped by the culture and training of surgeons.[9]

---

[9]This is underlined by the fact that attempts to introduce laparoscopy into general surgery for improving the diagnosis of acute appendicitis were not met with any great interest by the surgical community (Leape and Ramenofsky, 1980).

In very general terms, one might observe that patients often enter the specialized health care world through internal medicine and its subspecialties, and these specialties traditionally have spent a considerable time on diagnostic activities. As endoscopic tools entered the health care arena as diagnostic tools, they naturally fell into the hands of the internal medicine specialties, who subsequently were well-positioned in terms of training and skills to use endoscopes for therapeutic interventions. The surgical subspecialty that made extensive use of endoscopes was gynecology and obstetrics. Yet, over time gynecology has diminished considerably in importance in the general surgeon's training and practice (Gaskin et al., 1991). Moreover, the use of an endoscope essentially means that one operates outside of the patient's body, which in many ways was anathema to the culture of surgery. Generally speaking, surgeons are trained in a highly hierarchical community, where the teaching paradigm is passed on from one generation of surgeons to the next. In abdominal surgery, for example, the leading paradigm for recent generations of surgeons was to make large incisions that allowed them to directly visualize and palpate the abdomen and provided them with ample space to retract the liver and other organs, as necessary (interview with K. Reemstma, December 1991, chairman of surgery, Columbia University).

In the 1990s, the willingness of surgeons to adopt laparoscopy underwent dramatic change, as is probably most significantly illustrated in the case of gallstone surgery, which was the first major surgical procedure to be transformed into a laparoscopic procedure. Traditionally, gallstone disease has been defined as a surgical condition.[10]

The German surgeon Carl Langenbuch, surgeon-in-chief at the Lazarus Krankenhaus in Berlin, is generally credited with the first removal of the human gallbladder, or cholecystectomy, in 1882 (Langenbuch, 1882). With evolving surgical techniques and increasing experience, mortality and morbidity rates demonstrated an impressive decrease. By the end of the 1960s, cholecystectomy was widely regarded as a safe and effective procedure and, in essence, surgeons had a monopoly position in the treatment of gallstones.

In the 1970s this situation began to change. Gastroenterologists began to develop gallstone-dissolving drugs, as well as solvents that were percutaneously introduced into the gallbladder through an endoscope. An editorial in the *New England Journal of Medicine* indicated the emergence of interspecialty rivalries: "In the meantime our surgical colleagues can relax; their treatment of gallstones, although threatened, is not yet outmoded" (Isselbacher, 1972). Moreover, gastroenterologists, as described earlier, also successfully developed endoscopic removal of bile duct stones, as surgical intervention in the case of recurrent or retained common duct stones carried a significantly high mortality risk. Finally,

---

[10]At the end of the nineteenth century, surgeons first introduced cholecystostomy for stones in the gallbladder, and choledocholithotomy for stones in the bile duct. Cholecystectomy came to replace cholecystostomy as the operation of choice for gallstones.

and most importantly, in the mid-1980s, gastroenterologists and interventional radiologists introduced gallstone lithotripsy (originally developed for kidney stones). Although we now know that lithotripsy involves lengthy treatment periods, is applicable only to a minority of patients, has high costs, and carries a high risk of recurrence after successful treatment, at the time lithotripsy seemed to have a potential similar to that of tagamet and other H_2-blockers, which essentially led to the disappearance of ulcer surgery. These competitive pressures would be an important factor in inducing surgeons to develop laparoscopic cholecystectomy.

In March 1987, Philippe Mouret in Lyons, France, performed the first human laparoscopic cholecystectomy using a gynecological instrument. Concurrently, two centers in France and two in the United States began to further develop the technique (Dubois et al., 1989; Perissat, 1992; Reddick et al., 1989). As the laparoscope was similar to that used in gynecology, leading manufacturers of rigid endoscopes, such as Storz and Wolf, early on saw a major new opportunity and quickly capitalized on their technologies and reputations. In particular, their ability to provide add-on video cameras that could provide high-resolution realistic color images on a videomonitor was of utmost importance. Laparoscopic cholecystectomy generally involves three to four punctures and a team of three professionals inserting the necessary instruments into the abdomen, which underscores the importance of other members of the surgical team being able to observe the operation so that they can provide useful assistance. These clinicians also realized that applying surgical sutures through an endoscope was difficult and particularly time-consuming and would discourage a major part of the surgical profession from adopting the technique. The surgeons Reddick and Olsen worked together with U.S. Surgical, an existing wound closure company that more than 20 years ago developed a stapling device, to adapt this device for use through an endoscope. This achievement facilitated the application of laparoscopic cholecystectomy tremendously, and in the early 1990s U.S. Surgical became the dominant firm in this field. U.S. Surgical's leading position, however, is currently being contested by Johnson & Johnson's newly formed Ethicon Endo-Surgery division (Ethicon was the leading sutures manufacturer, making more than 80 percent of all sutures in the United States).

Finally, in European centers, the gallbladder itself was dissected from the liver by electrocautery devices, which had been available in all operating rooms since the 1960s. In the United States, laser companies were able to establish a link between their technologies and laparoscopic cholecystectomy. The application of lasers to laparoscopic cholecystectomy required major changes in the delivery of laser energy. Because CO_2 energy cannot be transmitted through endoscope fiber optics, CO_2 lasers were not useful. Laser companies, such as Coherent, Trimedyne, and Laserscope, developed argon, dual wave-length KTP, and contact yttrium-aluminum-garnet (YAG) lasers for use in laparoscopic cholecystectomies for which they sought FDA approval in 1989 and 1990 (Biomedical Business International, 1992).

These clinician-innovators and the industrial firms involved presented videotapes of the first laparoscopic cholecystectomy at surgical society meetings in 1989 (not during scientific sessions, but in the technical exhibition hall), and afterward the procedure underwent rapid diffusion, particularly in the United States. Table 4-1 shows the volume of laparoscopic and endoscopic procedures by specialty in 1991. A variety of factors played a role in the widespread adoption of the procedures by surgeons, including the above-mentioned provider competition. In addition, laparoscopic equipment received rapid regulatory approval because it was deemed "substantially equivalent" to the laparoscopes and soft-tissue lasers that were on the market before the 1976 Medical Device Amendments to the Food and Drug Act took effect. (Approval of the equipment was handled through a so-called 510[k] procedure rather than the full premarketing approval (PMA) review.) Moreover, payers supported use of the new technique because it promised significant cost savings. In addition, laparoscopic cholecystectomy was financially attractive to U.S. hospitals as they were reimbursed initially by Medicare at rates equal to conventional cholecystectomy. Relatively low start-up costs also contributed to diffusion: neither major changes in health care facilities nor large capital expenditures were required (unless a facility had to purchase a laser, which costs between $100,000 and $200,000). Last, but certainly not least, patient demand for the procedure was particularly high because it promised to be less painful, caused minimal scarring, and allowed earlier return to active life.

To accommodate the burgeoning demand, industry built commercial training

TABLE 4-1 Top 12 Laparoscopic or Endoscopic Procedures by Volume, 1991

Procedure	Specialist	1991
Esophagogastroduodenoscopy	Gastroenterologist	582,000
Colonoscopy	Gastroenterologist	272,000
Proctosigmoidoscopy	Gastroenterologist	240,000
Gastroenterologic biopsy	Gastroenterologist	240,000
Tubal ligation	Gynecologist	177,000
Cholecystectomy	General surgeon	127,000
Uterine adhesiolysis	Gynecologist	120,000
Gastroenterologic polypectomy	Gastroenterologist	64,000
Transurethral prostatectomy	Urologist	53,000
Gynecologic polypectomy	Gynecologist	64,000
Herniorrhaphy	General surgeon/urologist	45,000
Appendectomy	General surgeon	42,000

SOURCE: Biomedical Business International, 1991.

centers that provided hands-on experience in animals and simultaneously introduced surgeons to procedure-related products. With the introduction of commercial interests, the training process of surgeons in new procedures, which traditionally had been undertaken by other surgeons, underwent fundamental change. In the United States, more than 50 percent of the nation's 32,750 practicing general surgeons learned laparoscopic cholecystectomy during the 18 months after the procedure was introduced (White, 1991). Moreover, following the introduction of laparoscopic cholecystectomy, the pool of patients undergoing gallbladder removal expanded from sicker to mildly symptomatic patients (suggesting that this procedure is becoming at least partly prophylactic) as well as to higher-risk patients once considered ineligible for the procedure. As a result, the overall level of gallbladder removals increased (Legoretta et al., 1993). This means that, although laparoscopic cholecystectomies reduce unit costs by 25 percent (mostly because of shorter hospital stays), their introduction has resulted in an increase, not a decrease, in aggregate expenditures (Legoretta et al., 1993).

Adoption rates in Europe show a different trend: slower diffusion at half the rate seen in the United States. Several factors may account for the difference. One reason for this slower diffusion may be differences in payment mechanisms, especially in view of European reliance on hospital budgeting systems. In addition, European endoscope manufacturers, like Storz and Wolf, initially focused on the U.S. market and were unable to meet European demands for equipment. European restrictions on the use of animals for training purposes are another factor. These regulations require the use of operative simulators and observational methods, which can slow the time necessary to bring a surgeon to an adequate level of clinical competence (Biomedical Business International, 1992).

Rapidly escalating professional and patient demand for a less invasive way to remove gallstones precluded the performance of a controlled trial to establish the safety, efficacy, and indications for laparoscopic cholecystectomy. As a result, assessment relied on a large number of prospective case studies that reported equivalent patient outcomes in comparison to the open procedure. A greater number of serious procedure-related complications (e.g., bile duct injuries) were reported for laparoscopic cholecystectomy, but these seemed to be offset by the reported decreases in pain, co-morbidity-related complications (e.g., stroke, pulmonary embolism), hospital length of stay, and recovery period that resulted from the laparoscopic approach (Perissat and Vitale, 1991). For example, hospital length of stay decreased from four to six days to an overnight or ambulatory procedure; and return to work or normal activity decreased even more dramatically, from four to six weeks to less than one week (Southern Surgeons Club, 1991).

As with other surgical procedures, complication rates fell with operative experience. A "learning curve" for laparoscopic cholecystectomy has been well described, with rates of adverse events for an individual surgeon decreasing with operative experience. Laparoscopic cholecystectomy requires skill, dexterity, and the ability to perform surgery with a two-dimensional view of the patient's organs. It also requires coordination of hand motions that may appear reversed on the video monitor if the camera is directed at the surgeon. As a result of the often inadequate training of surgeons in this new technique, reports of surgical complications began to increase and cast a shadow over this new procedure. This led the state of New York to issue guidelines that require surgeons to perform at least 15 procedures under supervision before they can operate independently.

With the rapid dissemination of laparoscopic cholecystectomy came a large demand for the tools of the trade. All existing endoscope companies began to cater to the general surgeon and this sparked an unprecedented level of industrial competition both among existing endoscope manufacturers and new companies. In 1990, more than 80 companies had started to develop laparoscopy products. Along which lines did these companies compete? First, they put emphasis on developing a continuous stream of new and modified products (many of which are obsolete in as little as four to six months) and low-cost manufacturing methods. Second, the composition of R&D teams underwent considerable change. Ethicon Endo-Surgery, for example, quadrupled its engineering staff from 1989 levels. In their quest to develop new instruments, companies began to work more closely and earlier in the development process with surgeons they consider thought-leaders or innovators. Several firms also have added surgeons to their in-house R&D teams, and have started to provide their engineers with clinical training. Moreover, as the possibility of integrating minimally invasive devices with biologicals emerges on the technological horizon, some firms are extending their R&D teams in the direction of molecular biologists. Finally, a dynamic pattern of interindustry alliances, acquisitions, and mergers is emerging. For example, Olympus and Ethicon Endo-Surgery signed a cooperative agreement to share R&D, marketing, and particularly training programs, whereas the camera firm Cabot Medical merged with the electrocautery manufacturer Birtcher to become a full-line supplier of products.

Moving from the rate to the direction of development, manufacturers are still now focusing on improving the ease of device operation by developing improved organ extractors and trocars, robotic arms, and modified suture applicators. Moreover, camera manufacturers are focusing on improving visualization and clarity by incorporating new chip technology into their cameras, as well as monitoring advances in high-definition television for its application in medical video imaging. Furthermore, the ongoing conversion of other traditionally open surgical procedures, such as hernia repair, vagotomy, appendectomies, colon surgery, and bowel resection, to laparoscopic procedures is leading to the demand for new instrumentation. Bowel resection, for example, requires larger instruments to be passed through the laparoscope which, in turn, requires large operating channels. The conversion of these procedures is, however, occurring much less rapidly than was the case with laparoscopic cholecystectomy. This slower diffusion process is a result of the recognized need for special training, the longer operating room time involved in these laparoscopic procedures, and the more recent reluctance of payers to cover these procedures because of the possibility of expansions of use (Halter, 1994).

Finally, increasing competition among suppliers has meant that price and operating costs are beginning to play a role in decisions about development targets. For example, in the early stages of use of laparoscopic cholecystectomy, lasers were preferred over electrocautery as the gallbladder dissection method of choice in the United States. Large case series comparing the two techniques demonstrated that both were safe and effective, but electrocautery was shown to be less expensive and is now used in the majority of cases (Southern Surgeons Club, 1991). Another issue has been whether to focus on the development of reusable or disposable products. In Europe, the emphasis has been on improving reusable devices, as a result of concerns over equipment cost and toxic waste disposal, which tend to be stronger there than in the United States. Wolf, for instance, has developed a reusable trocar that can be easily resharpened. The U.S. firms, particularly U.S. Surgical and Ethicon, focused on disposable instruments, arguing that disposables protected against cross-infections and did not require the time and costs of sterilization and repackaging. Reusable instruments manufacturers countered these charges by arguing that reusables were more cost-effective, and the disposable manufacturers now increasingly started to compete on the basis of price. U.S. Surgical, for example, announced at the 1992 American College of Surgeons meeting that it would bring a disposable laparoscope to the market for less than $200.

SOME CONCLUDING OBSERVATIONS AND SPECULATIONS

First, some brief observations about the nature of the interdisciplinary relationship in endoscopy. This chapter indicates that endoscopic innovation has indeed been highly dependent on scientific and engineering advances that are generated outside of the medical sector, such as fiber optics, color television, and charge couple devices. This characteristic has important implications for the timing of innovation: it means, for example, that the realization of the first endoscope—which had been conceptualized already in the Middle Ages—and subsequent modifications of existing equipment had to await advances in areas of science and technology over which the medical profession had little to no control. Yet we are oversimplifying a complex and subtle relationship if we picture medicine merely as a passive receiver. In the case of fiber optics, for instance, attempts by Hirschowitz, Curtiss, and Peters to develop a flexible GI endoscope led them to solve two major problems that properly belonged to the realm of physics and engineering: (a) by coating the fibers with glass of a lower refractive index they successfully addressed the critical problem of "cross talk," and (b) they created a novel process for manufacturing aligned flexible fiber bundles. Thus, certain key manufacturing problems, which had to be resolved before fiber optics could obtain its widespread industrial usage, were first addressed in the academic/medical community, not the industrial community. These advances, in turn, made an important contribution to optical physics research and the eventual application of fiber optics and endoscopes in other sectors of the economy, such as telecommunications, but also the defense and aircraft industries. In sum, fiber optics, a major medical innovation, not only came into the world through medical instrumentation, but the medical world itself made significant contributions to the *advancement* of that technology. As Kapany observes: "From a historical viewpoint, the very origin of fiber optics is intimately linked with its application in medicine."

Given the inherently interdisciplinary nature of endoscopic innovation, it is not surprising that close interactions between user clinicians and industrial firms, often in academic medical centers, were found to be crucial to the successful development of medical technology. These interactions are important for a variety of reasons that move beyond the stylized view of the division of labor between academic and industrial settings. This oversimplified view may be summarized in the following manner: Clinicians in universities undertake biomedical research and provide feedback about the shortcomings of technologies when introduced into clinical practice; this knowledge then leads industry to develop and manufacture new and improved technologies. Whereas the behavior of clinicians who adopt or reject certain technologies over time has indeed fed back important signals to industrial firms about the kinds of projects that may be worthwhile to undertake, our study material suggests that the medical profession also plays a more active role in the development of new products. The majority of endoscopic innovations considered in this analysis are user dominated, in the sense that clinicians were instrumental in designing and developing the prototype and not merely in articulating the need for some specific new instrument. However, and perhaps more unexpectedly, the medical/academic world in certain cases (e.g., the development of the first flexible fiberscope) also solved what in essence were a set of manufacturing problems and provided expertise about the scaling up for production to the industrial firm—activities normally thought of as the proper domain of the manufacturing sector.

Our study points to an additional, and quite significant, finding, and that is that the existing disciplinary boundaries *internal* to medicine itself may have constituted an even more serious obstacle to innovation than those external to medicine. Put somewhat differently, the most difficult barriers that needed to be crossed were not between medicine and industry, but barriers within medicine itself. For example, the transfer of laparoscopy from gynecology to surgery seems to have taken an unnecessarily long time. Whereas this lag may be partially explained by the fact that more complex surgical procedures had to await the introduction of complementary technologies (such as video endoscopy), this alone does not appear to provide a satisfactory explanation. The delay in transfer appears to be intimately linked to issues surrounding the definition and the boundaries of clinical specialties. As mentioned, internal medicine and its sub-specialties, such as gastroenterology, have traditionally borne primary responsibility for diagnostic activities, and endoscopic tools were part and parcel of the culture and training of these specialties. The adoption of flexible endoscopic procedures by gastroenterologists and other internists was generally rapid, particularly in those cases—such as colonoscopy—where the new procedure did not displace an older procedure with vested interests. By contrast, recent generations of surgeons had little training in endoscopic procedures, and, as described above, laparoscopy was in many ways contrary to the culture of surgery. Indeed, for many decades surgeons were not particularly interested in the adoption of surgical laparoscopy. Starting in 1989, however, the attitudes of surgeons underwent major change, and—as mentioned—in the United States more than half of all general surgeons acquired the necessary skills within 18 months, a breathtakingly rapid adoption of a new medical procedure by any historical standard. It is interesting to note that this adoption process was, at least in part, a generational phenomenon. Preliminary evidence of a major study by the American College of Surgeons indicates that younger surgeons, who lacked the lifelong investment in the older procedure, were more willing to invest the time and take the risks involved in adopting laparoscopic cholecystectomy.

How can we reconcile the apparently conservative attitude of surgeons throughout most of the previous decades with this sudden switch in the 1990s? Although strong demand by patients and payers for less invasive and less costly procedures certainly was an important factor, and a factor that became more important over time, our study suggests the possibility that interspecialty competition may well have played the dominant role. In particular, the development and introduction of gallstone lithotripsy by gastroenterologists and interventional radiologists during the mid-1980s appeared to pose an important threat to the position of surgeons in the treatment of gallstone disease. These competitive pressures, compounded by a growing concern over health care costs (see below), induced surgeons to adopt and further develop laparoscopic cholecystectomy, which subsequently has effectively challenged the then-perceived advantages of biliary lithotripsy.

The adoption of laparoscopy by the surgical profession led to a high level of industrial innovation and competition, as indicated by the entry of new firms into the market and the continuous stream of new products. This competitive environment also stimulated a stronger focus on interdisciplinary R&D than in earlier times. For example, in previous decades industrial firms, such as Storz, had consultancy arrangements with leading clinicians, such as the gynecologist Semm. Nowadays, these consultancy arrangements are still important, but a new arrangement for piercing disciplinary boundaries is becoming apparent: the composition of the R&D team is undergoing significant change in that surgeons are becoming part of the in-house R&D team and engineers are receiving more extensive clinical training. The academic-industry interface is also changing in other ways: for the first time in the history of surgery industry has become actively involved in *teaching* these new procedures. At this point, it seems important to emphasize the industrial experience with these technologies: new technologies once introduced into the world often take on a subsequent life of their own. Commercial success or failure turns upon considerations of a very different sort than those we have considered so far. For example, many of the original rigid GI endoscope manufacturers failed to make the discontinuous leap to a world of fiber optics and were driven out of the industry. ACMI, a leader in the early development of flexible fiber-optic endoscopes, subsequently lost its market position to Japanese producers (just like the Eder Instrument Company with the sigmoidoscope). Indeed, Olympus now controls 75 percent of the world market in gastroenterological endoscopy. It appears that the conditions determining eventual *commercial success* with new technologies may be very different from those determining success in making the *initial innovation*. As a conjecture, Olympus's success would appear to result from its unique strengths in both sales and after-sales service and maintenance, as well as from its flexibility and speed in responding to user needs.

The issues of interspecialty and interindustry competition are, in turn, closely linked to changes that are presently occurring in the delivery and financing of health care. In the 1980s, attempts to control the rising costs took on a new urgency, and are leading to major changes in the payment system and the incentives incorporated in this system. This has affected the rate, but also the direction, of technological change. The direction in which industrial developers try to move their technologies is embodied in their selection of R&D projects. In the period before these constraints came into play, judgments by the relevant medical specialty about a technology's clinical performance have predominated in determining the directions in which improvements are sought, and feedback signals are often couched in terms of shortcomings in the efficacy and safety of existing treatment options. Problems involving the ease of operation of the technology for professionals or the quality of care for patients have been another important influence. Yet, in the case of surgical laparoscopy the first signs (e.g., the debate on reusables versus disposables, or the emerging preferences for electrocautery over lasers) are appearing that economic considerations will increasingly influence the direction of technological change in the years to come.

These preliminary conclusions suggest an agenda for future research. First on this agenda is the matter of interspecialty competition. Whereas the economics literature has extensively debated the ways in which competition among industrial developers may affect the pace of generating and developing new technologies, there is no discussion in the literature of the phenomenon of competition among *user groups*. A careful examination of the effects of interspecialty competition on the rate and direction of technological change may be a fruitful area of further research. The second issue, in these times of health care reform, concerns how new incentives might be introduced to deal with the tension between cost containment on the one hand and medical innovation on the other. How can we devise financial incentives to induce the medical-industrial world to develop cost-reducing new technologies? This is not—yet—a well-formulated question because the impact of a new medical technology on health care costs is not something that is intrinsic in a piece of hardware, such as an endoscope. It will depend also upon the sort of *use* that the medical profession choses to make of that hardware, and those choices will also be shaped by the prevailing payment system. These are issues that have yet to be examined.

REFERENCES

Anderson, E. T. 1937. Peritoneoscopy. *American Journal of Surgery* 35:36–39.

Berci, G., Adler, D. A., Brooks, P. G., Pasternak, A., and Hasler, G. 1973. The importance of instrumentation and documentation in gynecological laparoscopy. *Journal of Reproductive Medicine* 10:276–284.

Berci, G., and Davids, J. 1962. Endoscopy and television. *British Medical Journal* 1:1610–1613.

Berci, G., Adler, D., Brooks, P. G., Pasternak, A., and Hasler, G. 1973. The importance of instrumentation and documentation in gynecological laparoscopy. *Journal of Reproductive Medicine* 10:276–284.

Biomedical Business International. 1992. U.S. market for products in laparoscopic/endoscopic surgery. Santa Ana, Calif.

Classen, M., and Demling, L. 1974. Endoskopische Sphincterotomie der Papilla Vateri und Steinextraktion aus dem Ductus Choledocus. *Deutsche Medische Wochenschrifte* 99:496–497.

Classen, M., and Phillip, J. 1984. Electronic endoscopy of the gastrointestinal tract: Initial experience with a new type of endoscope that has a new fiberoptic bundle for imaging. *Endoscopy* 16:16–19.

Dubois, F., Berthelot, G., and Levard, H. 1989. Cholécystectomy par coelioscopy. *Nouvelle Presse Medicale* 18:980–982.

Filipi, C. J., Fitzgibbons, R. J., and Salerno, G. M. 1991. Historical review: Diagnostic laparoscopy to laparoscopic cholecystectomy and beyond. In: K. A. Zucker, ed. *Surgical Laparoscopy*. St. Louis: Quality Medical Publishing, pp. 3–21.

Fourestier, M., Gladu, A., and Vulmière, J. 1952. Perfectionnements à l'endoscopie médicale. Réalisation bronchoscopique. *La Presse Médicale* 60:1292–1294.

Gaskin, T. A., Isobe, J. H., Mathews, J. L., Winchester, S. B., and Smith, R. J. 1991. Laparoscopy and the general surgeon. *Surgical Clinics of North America* 71:1085–1097.

Gunning, J. E. 1974. The history of laparoscopy. In: *Gynecological Laparoscopy: Principles and Techniques.* J. M. Phillips and L. Keith, eds. New York: Stratton Intercontinental Medical Books, pp. 57–66.

Halter, P. 1994. Minimally invasive surgery. *Medical Device & Diagnostic Industry* (January):68–72.

Haubrich, W. S. 1987. History of endoscopy. In: *Gastroenterologic Endoscopy*. M. V. Sivak, ed. Philadelphia: W. B. Saunders.

Hirschowitz, B. I. 1961. Endoscopic examination of the stomach and duodenal cap with the fiberscope. *Lancet* 1:1074–1078.

Hirschowitz, B. I. 1979. A personal history of the fiberscope. *Gastroenterology* 76:864–869.

Hirschowitz, B. I. 1989. The fibre-optic era in endoscopy—beginnings and perspectives. *Italian Journal of Gastroenterology* 21:247–250.

Hopkins, H. H., and Kapany, N. S. 1954. A flexible fiberscope, using static scanning. *Nature* 17:39–41.

Hulka, J. F., Fishburne, J. I., Mercer, J. P., et al. 1973. Laparoscopic sterilization with a spring-loaded clip: A report on the first fifty cases. *American Journal of Obstetrics and Gynecology* 116:715.

Isselbacher, K. J. 1972. A medical treatment for gallstones? *New England Journal of Medicine* 286:40–42.

Kalk, H. 1929. Erfahrungen mit der Laparoskopie. *Zeitschrift fur Klinische Medizin* 14:303.

Kawai, K., Akasaka, Y., Murakinu, K., et al. 1974. Endoscopic sphincterotomy of the ampulla of Vater. *Gastrointestinal Endoscopy* 20:148–151.

Kodama, F. 1992. Technology fusion and the new R&D. *Harvard Business Review*, July-August, pp. 70–78.

Langenbuch, C. 1882. Ein Fall von Exstirpation der Gallenblase wegen chronischer cholelithiasis: Heilung. *Berliner Klinische Wochenschrift* 19:725–727.

Leape, L., and Ramenofsky, M. L. 1980. Laparoscopy for questionable appendicitis. *Annals of Surgery* 191:400–413.

Legoretta, A.P., et al. 1993. Increased cholecystectomy rate after the introduction of laparoscopic cholecystectomy. *Journal of the American Medical Association* 270:1429–1432.

Liskin, L., Rinehart, W., Blackburn, R., and Rutledge, A. H. 1985. Female sterilization. *Population Reports* 9:128–129.

Oi, I., Kobayashi, S., and Koudo, T. 1970. Endoscopic pancreatocholangiography. *Endoscopy* 2:103-106.

Overholt, B. F. 1981. The history of colonoscopy. In: *Colonoscopy Techniques*. R. H. Hunt and J. D. Waye, eds. London: Chapman and Hall.

Palmer, R. 1947. Instrumentation et technique de la coelioscopie gynécologique. *Gynecologie et Obstetrie* (Paris) 46:420–431.

Palmer, R. 1962. Essais de sterilisation tuballe coelioscopique par electrocoagulation isthmique. *Bulletin de la Féderation des Sociétiés de Gynecologie et d'Obstetrique de Langue Française* 14:298–301.

Perissat, J. 1992. Laparoscopic Cholecystectomy—The European Experience. Presentation at the Consensus Development Conference, National Institutes of Health, Bethesda, Md., September 14–16.

Perissat, J., and Vitale, G. C. 1991. Laparoscopic cholecystectomy: Gateway to the future. *American Journal of Surgery* 161:408.

Perna, G., Honda, T., and Morrissey, J. 1965. Gastrocamera photography. *Archives of Internal Medicine* 116:434–444.

Reddick, E. J., Olsen, D., Daniell, J., Saye, W., et al. 1989. Laparoscopic laser cholecystectomy. *Laser Medical and Surgical News Advances* (February):38–40.

Rioux, J. E. 1989. Female sterilization and its reversal. In: *Contraception: Science and Practice*. M. Filshie and J. Guilleband, eds. London: Butterworths, pp. 275–291.

Rioux, J. E., and Cloutier, D. 1974. A new bipolar instrument for laparoscopic tubal sterilization. *American Journal of Obstetrics and Gynecology* 119:737–739.

Salmon, P.R. 1974. *Fibre-optic Endoscopy*. New York: Pittman Medical Publishing Co. pp. 4–5.

Semm, K. 1977. *Atlas of Gynecologic Laparoscopy and Hysteroscopy*. Philadelphia: W. B. Saunders.

Semm, K. 1987. *Operative Manual for Endoscopic Abdominal Surgery*. Chicago: Year Book Medical Publishers.

Shinya, H. 1982. *Colonoscopy: Diagnosis and Treatment of Colonic Diseases*. Tokyo: Igaku-Shoin, p. v.

Soulas, A. 1956. Television bronchologie et pneumologie. *La Presse Médicale* 64:97–99.

Southern Surgeons Club. 1991. A prospective analysis of 1,518 laparoscopic cholecystectomies. *New England Journal of Medicine* 324:1073–1078.

Steptoe, P. C. 1967. *Laparoscopy in Gynecology*. Edinburgh: Livingstone.

van Heel, A. C. S. 1954. A new method of transporting optical images without aberrations. *Nature* 17:39.

Wheeless, C. R., Jr. 1972. Elimination of second incision in laparoscopic sterilization. *Obstetrics and Gynecology* 39:134–136.

White, J. V. 1991. Laparoscopic cholecystectomy: The evolution of general surgery. *Annals of Internal Medicine* 115:651–653.

Wildegans, H. 1960. *Die Operative Gallengangsendoskopie*. Munchen: Urban and Schwarzenberg.

Wortman, J., and Piotrow, P. T. 1973. Colpotomy: The vaginal approach. *Population Reports* 3:29–44.

Yoon, J. B., and King, T. M. 1975. A preliminary and intermediate report on a new laparoscopic tubal ring procedure. *Journal of Reproductive Medicine* 15:54–56.

5

Cochlear Implantation:
Establishing Clinical Feasibility, 1957–1982

STUART S. BLUME

THE IDEA OF ELECTRICAL STIMULATION
OF THE HUMAN EAR

Between the second half of the nineteenth century and World War II, a gap opened up between the scientific investigation of hearing on the one hand and the clinical (sub)specialty concerned with the ear—otology—on the other (Bordley and Brookhouser, 1979). For decades, the principal concern of otologists was with the (surgical) treatment of diseased tissue in and around the organ of hearing. Otologic surgeons developed many procedures designed to correct malfunctioning in the middle ear (fenestration, tympanoplasty) and in the vestibular system which provides the human with a sense of balance. Meanwhile, building on Helmholtz's classic studies, research on the nature and mechanisms of hearing was being conducted by physiologists, psychologists, and physicists. It was only rarely, and perhaps only in major centers of scholarship and research, that otologists were involved in this work.

In 1930, Wever and Bray, working in the Department of Experimental Psychology at Princeton University, discovered the so-called "cochlear microphonic potential." They showed that if electrical contact was made with the auditory nerve of a cat and the potentials developed in it were amplified and passed through telephone receivers, sounds delivered to the animal's ear could be recognized by a listener. The quality of the "cat microphone" was such that if words were spoken into the cat's ear, a remote listener could identify them through the receiver. Although electrical phenomena were already known to be involved in the mechanism of hearing, this finding had major theoretical implications and it generated considerable interest (Davis, 1935). Various theories were put forward about how exactly mechanical vibrations (sound waves) are turned into electrical stimuli carried by the auditory nerve to the brain. The inner ear, or cochlea, functioned as a transducer. But how, exactly? And what components of its complex structure were involved? Most of this research was conducted on experimental animals: cats and guinea pigs. Gradually, in the course of the 1930s and 1940s, connections between this work and another well-known but curious fact began to be made. In 1800, Alessandro Volta had passed an electrical current through his head by placing an electrode, connected to a battery, in each ear. Completing the circuit led to a disagreeable sensation and a noise said to have been like the boiling of thick soup. Some subsequent experiments failed to replicate Volta's finding. In the 1930s, a number of workers were investigating this phenomenon, that is, the generation of acoustic effects by electrical stimulation of the ear. A particularly active group was at Harvard University: S. S. Stevens (Psychology Laboratory), H. Davis (Department of Physiology, Harvard Medical School), and M. H. Lurie (Department of Otology, Harvard Medical School). A series of experiments was carried out, along the following lines. Electrical circuits were made in which one electrode was a copper wire inserted into a saline-filled ear, while the ground electrode was attached to the arm. Various AC and DC currents were used. Depending upon characteristics of the circuit and the ear, various acoustic sensations could be induced in an experimental subject: a pure tone corresponding to the frequency of an alternating current; a "buzzing" noise independent of frequency; both tone and noise; or (in some listeners) nothing at all. Tones tended to be distorted. Stevens demonstrated this by connecting the electrodes of the subject to the output circuit of a radio:

> Music can be heard and popular tunes identified, but the quality is definitely poor—"tin pan" music. Speech can easily be recognized as speech, but only occasional words can be understood. Clearly, electrical stimulation does not promise much as an alternative means of hearing so long as so much distortion is present (Stevens, 1937).

In 1940, it was hypothesized that this electrophonic phenomenon takes place by three distinctive mechanisms (Jones et al., 1940). One of these mechanisms, the one generating the pure tone, was believed to be related to the cochlear microphonic, in which a vibration was thought to be set up in an intracochlear membrane. The noise phenomenon was believed to be due to direct stimulation of the auditory nerve, a result also obtained by workers in the Soviet Union (Andreef et al., 1935). A "threshold effect" was also noted. Small differences in voltage separated an acoustic sensation from the experience of pain. Moreover, because the auditory nerve is also involved in the sense of balance, and also lies very close to the facial nerve, dizziness or facial twitches could also ensue.

With the emergence of modern audiology, concerned with the clinical assessment of hearing in the 1940s and 1950s, and the subsequent development of sophisticated audiometric devices, the focus of general otological practice began to change. Through an emergent partnership with audiology (which in many European countries—in contrast to America and Britain—emerged as a specialization within medical otology) otologists were beginning to develop a new interest in hearing. Many of their older preoccupations, like lupus, were of declining significance, thanks to new antibiotics (Jongkees, 1982). Nevertheless, in the 1950s and 1960s interventions were still limited to addressing (typically mechanical) deficiencies of the middle ear. Problems of the inner ear, associated with so-called sensorineural deafness, remained intractable. There was nothing in current practice, either surgical intervention or in the acoustic amplification provided by a conventional hearing aid, that offered hearing to the sensorineurally deaf. This was so despite continuing work in neurophysiology and psychophysics, which was adding to understanding of basic mechanisms.

In February 1957, a totally deaf person about to be operated on begged Paris otologist C. Eyries to try to give him some minimal hearing. Eyries approached A. Djourno, who was working on electrical stimulation of the auditory nerve in animals. After some deliberation they decided to try to implant the patient with an electrode, similar to that used in the animal research, which would stimulate his (functioning) auditory nerve. The electrode was constructed in the physics laboratory of the University of Paris Faculty of Medicine, and on February 25, 1957, this device was implanted. Various tests were done, but in March the device broke down. It was repaired and replanted, and in July rehabilitation was started with a speech therapist. Very rapidly the patient's initial enthusiasm faded, as his expectations failed to be borne out. It soon became apparent to the patient that different kinds of sounds could not be distinguished: speech, opening a door, dragging a chair—all sounded the same. In March 1958, the patient decided that he wanted to terminate the rehabilitation. Nevertheless, despite the bulk of the device and despite the difficulties in distinguishing frequencies (which suggested to them that more than one electrode would be needed), Eyries and Djourno felt that the technique had a future. The three cases they implanted between February 1957 and November 1958 gave cause for optimism, they felt (Albinhac, 1978; Djourno and Eyries, 1957).

A Los Angeles otologist, William House, was one of those inspired by a report of this work. Then of the Ear Research Institute in Los Angeles, "an ordinary ear doctor," he was intrigued by what Djourno and Eyries had tried to achieve:

> I remember that a patient brought me a little clipping from a newspaper about this particular work and about the results on the patient. That was in my first year of practice, which was 1956. I was very stimulated by that. I thought it was amazing that this might be done. I went ahead and got the article and had it translated because I don't read French very well. The amazing thing to me is that Djourno and Eyries never published any more on it, nor did they do more than, I think, two patients. That stimulated a lot of interest on my part. I remember getting some oscillators and electrodes together and during the stapes

and chronic ear surgery we were doing at that time . . . we had a lot of opportunities to put electrodes on the promontory during surgery and ask the patients what they heard. It was really an eye opener what they could hear from these electrical stimulations during surgery.

This encouraged us then to pick out some patients who had total losses as volunteers, and take them to surgery and try some of these stimulations . . . (House, 1985).

In 1961, House implanted an electrode, constructed by a collaborating engineer, into the cochlea (more precisely, the scala tympani) of a man deaf from advanced otosclerosis. House's implant was different from that used in Paris. It was designed so as to stimulate the cochlea at five different positions along its length. The electrode was soon rejected. The wires were insulated with silicone rubber which at that time contained some toxic substances. The implanted patient began to develop symptoms that led Dr. House to explant the electrode after about three weeks. In addition, recalls House,

we were also beset by other problems. We began to be deluged by calls from people who had heard about the implant and its possibilities. The engineer who had constructed the implant exercised bad judgment and encouraged newspaper articles about the research we were doing. We brought the first phase of our active investigations to a halt (House and Urban, 1973).

In fact, the engineer who had been working with Dr. House formed a company intended to sell stock in what was later to become the House implant. It is noteworthy that, although Dr. House dissolved the partnership, the engineer in question was able to continue work on the subject with another group in Los Angeles. They published what was probably the very first U.S. paper on the subject in 1963 (Doyle et al., 1963). Although convinced of the potential of the technique, Dr. House suspended active work on cochlear implantation at this point.

Blair Simmons, professor in the department of otolaryngology at Stanford Medical School, came to cochlear implantation with a quite different set of interests and resources. Simmons had a long-standing scientific interest in physiological processes of sound and pitch reception. In the 1950s, he had been involved in experimental work involving placing electrodes in the entrance to the cochlea (the so-called "round window") using cats. Like Eyries and Djourno earlier, Simmons was presented with the opportunity to attempt something on a human (who had nothing to lose) which he had previously (only) tried on experimental animals. Simmons carried out his first experiment with a patient who had had a right cerebelectomy in 1962 (Simmons et al., 1964). Part of the rationale was to see if the patient could adequately distinguish pitch on the basis of differences in the rate of stimulation. Then-current theory suggested that so-called "rate encoding" should be possible, but only to a small extent. He subsequently wrote of this work:

We had the unexpected opportunity to stimulate the auditory nerve under direct vision in a patient who had previously had a right cerebelectomy. It seemed like an interesting thing to do even though nearly everyone who was an authority on hearing was then firmly convinced that Wever's and other earlier volley theories were totally wrong. It was thought that if the rate pitch did exist it was limited to no more than 200 Hz—the buzz and cricket sounds described by Djourno and Eyries in 1957, and by others in the 1930s (Simmons, 1985).

It appeared from first observations that this patient perceived much more than would theoretically have been expected:

> It seemed reasonable to repeat these stimulations with better controls. By this time my animal work with electrodes had long since left the round window in favor of recording via permanent electrodes in the scala tympani and the modiolus. While insertion of these electrodes did produce serious tissue damage in about one-half of the animals, many were without damage. . . . It seemed reasonable to use these same methods with a human volunteer (Simmons, 1985).

Simmons was also *provoked*, he says, by the 1963 publication, which had made him very angry with its (in his view) "irresponsible claims" that the deaf could be made to hear (interview with F. B. Simmons, Stanford University, April 20, 1992). In May 1964, Simmons and a Stanford colleague implanted a 6-electrode array into the modiolus of a 60-year-old volunteer subject who was totally deaf in the right ear and was losing his hearing in the left ear. Suffering from retinitis pigmentosa, the subject was also losing his sight. "We were amazingly lucky," Blair Simmons commented later. "All electrodes functioned and remained so until he was explanted 18 months later" (Simmons, 1985). The subject could identify sound as speech by recognizing low sound frequencies, the time patterns, and some variation in loudness, but he could not identify individual words or phrases. The paper in which Simmons (1965) reported this work, published in *Science*, recounts a series of experiments done with this subject. Many of these experiments concern the subject's ability to discriminate stimuli that differed either in the location of the electrode stimulated ("place encoding") or in the number of pulses per second provided ("rate encoding").

The *participation* of the subject in this research is itself worthy of note: he is presented as a virtual co-worker (see Simmons et al., 1965).[1] The named co-workers, however, are not from California but from Bell Telephone Laboratories in New Jersey. Simmons had been unable to find local experts in auditory psychophysics willing to work with him in confirming the kinds of results he was getting with his 60-year old subject. It so happened that one of his graduate

---

[1]The subject appears in the paper as literally contributing through his own informed judgment ("The comparison with a bee buzz offered by the subject seemed particularly informative"; "judging from the subject's description of the sounds . . ."). This corresponds with Fox's account of clinician-subject relations in transplant programs (see Fox and Swazey, 1974).

students knew people at the Bell lab in Orange, New Jersey. They were very interested in doing the verification, provided Simmons was willing to assume full responsibility for the patient. "They were outsiders. I don't think they'd read the publicity" (interview with F. B. Simmons, Stanford University, April 20, 1992). Legal liability for the patient was also something: neither Bell nor Stanford University was willing to accept it. Simmons and his wife traveled with the patient who, 60 and nearly blind, was making his first trip by plane. At the Bell labs they got the same results, and this resulted in the *Science* paper of 1965.

The scientific and medical communities were not persuaded by the results that Simmons obtained. The American Otological Society rejected presentation of this work at their 1965 meeting, while an application for funding to the National Institutes of Health (NIH) was turned down. Blair Simmons then stopped working on human auditory stimulation, though continuing with related experimental work on cats.

By the 1960s, many investigators had produced acoustic sensations by means of electrical stimulation of the inner ear, in the context of research into the nature of hearing. Whatever the long-term objectives or expectations of these studies might have been, no one previously had sought to carry out such work in a clinical context. The clinical context had previously been, as it were, *latent.* We can see traces of it in, for example, Stevens' observation (quoted above) that in the present state of things "electrical stimulation does not promise much as an alternative means of hearing" (Stevens, 1937). It could, however, be invoked where the constraints of scientific argumentation were removed, for example, in newspaper accounts. The slightest suggestion of "making the deaf hear" was enough. M. H. Lurie, in a 1973 discussion, refers to the work that he and others had carried out in the 1930s:

> I remember when Dr. Davis and I gave the first demonstration at the international meeting of the Physiologists. The newspapers obtained a report of the presentation. The first thing I knew I received letters from individuals all over the world asking when could they come and have their hearing restored and that is the great danger of . . . this work appearing in the newspapers and the ensuing publicity. . . . There will be people demanding that these procedures be done on them . . . (Lurie, 1973).

Eyries and Djourno, House, and Simmons had now made the clinical context of electrical stimulation *manifest.* However, it is clear that at that time artificial stimulation within a clinical context could not be sustained. House, Eyries, and Simmons each stopped work after two or three attempts, discouraged by the recalcitrance of both the communities and the materials with which they had to work. Neither technology nor professional communities could support their ambitions. Within a few years, however, both House and Simmons were drawn back to the idea of the clinical application of electrical stimulation to humans. What led them to start again?

House, who started again in 1968, refers to technical developments: in materials technology resulting from the development of heart pacemakers, as well as in electronics (the transistor). Blair Simmons, who resumed work in 1971, explains the developments that led him to do so not in terms of advances in available technology, but in terms of the willingness of technologists (and physiologists) to collaborate with him. In the 1960s, there had been problems he had not been able to overcome:

> Gaining credibility or even cooperation from scientific colleagues in 1964 was not easy, particularly in California. The basic scientists were openly hostile towards anything having to do with cochlear implants, largely because there were extravagant claims for implants being made, both at clinical meetings and in the newspapers. Speech was said to be understood. Some patients could even converse over the telephone. There were testimonials about hearing the chirping of mockingbirds once again, enjoying symphony music, etc.
>
> While my 1964–1965 experiments were in progress I contacted at least six of the most prominent researchers in speech coding and others in auditory psychophysics. None of these persons were willing or interested in suggesting experiments which might have helped define speech coding strategies for the future. I got a distinct impression, perhaps colored by a little personal paranoia after the first few rejections, that everyone was either incapable of thinking about the many problems involved or would rather not risk tainting their scientific careers . . . (Simmons, 1985).

In the course of time, he recounts, he "learned the hard way that this type of experimentation needs a team. . . . It was and is easy to place electrodes in ears. The hard part is deciding upon coding schemes and the hardware and software to stimulate these electrodes" (Simmons, 1985).

In contrast to the situation in the early sixties, work in the seventies *could* be sustained. Not only House and Simmons, but San Francisco colleague Robin Michelson, followed by otologists across the United States, Europe (Austria, Britain, France, Germany, and Switzerland), and Australia, involved themselves in cochlear implantation. By about 1980, their efforts had led to the stabilization of a clinical context for this work. Otologists were beginning to accept that cochlear implantation had a place in professional practice, and industry was beginning to manifest some interest. The stage was being set for a complex debate, in which, for some, cochlear implantation would come to "stand for" a medical understanding of deafness which they increasingly rejected. Ethical, social, scientific, educational, and economic arguments, interests, and perspectives became inextricably interwoven in a bitter debate, which still continues. In this paper the perspective is more limited. The empirical focus here is on some of the programs of work on implantation that flourished in the 1970s. Analytically, we shall try to understand how these workers, collectively, sought to establish the clinical context within which cochlear implantation could eventually become an acceptable medical treatment for sensorineural deafness. As we look at these programs of work we shall see that they differ in fundamental respects from one another. Another question to be addressed then, will be why and how they differ. By the way of reaching answers to these questions, we will first make some general observations about how approaches to implementation may differ and then review in some detail the new beginnings made in cochlear implantation during the 1970s. We shall then be in a position to characterize how the process of establishing clinical feasibility unfolded and, finally, draw conclusions.

APPROACHES TO IMPLANTATION

The argument developed in *Insight and Industry* is that the "career" of a new medical technology is highly dependent on whether it emerges within or outside an existing "inter-organizational field" (Blume, 1992). That is, when the "vision" of a new technology emerges within an existing field of relationships between professionals and their supplying industry, it is sustained by existing structures. Work on the new modality can be published in established journals, attracts an established audience, and can be assessed on the basis of agreed criteria of utility and according to established research protocols. By contrast, a conception emerging outside such a field faces quite different sorts of problems. For whom is it of interest? How is its value to be assessed? How can the expertise necessary for its further elaboration be assembled? In these terms, and given the lack of prior clinical approaches to sensorineural deafness, we would expect the development of cochlear implantation to pose major problems of assembling the necessary human resources. And so it seems to have been. Pioneers in the field who may have agreed about little else nevertheless agree that it was an uphill battle. They faced considerable direct opposition in the early years, particularly from *within* the scientific community.

Far more was—and is—needed than the skills of the surgeon. At the very least, a program of cochlear implantation requires a device (so that both electrodes and speech processors have to be developed and built, a task for electronics experts); it requires subjects (who of necessity have to believe that the uncertain benefits of an experimental procedure are worth the physical and emotional costs); and it requires a means of teaching implantees to make sense of the unfamiliar acoustic sensations which they receive (which may require the skills of a speech therapist). The essentially interdisciplinary nature of cochlear implant development reflects the problems of assembling these, and perhaps other, skills and integrating their contributions.

A review of work on the emerging technique published in 1978 draws attention to the range of problems which cochlear implantation still posed:

> Artificial stimulation of the auditory system therefore poses difficult problems for the surgeon, the engineer, the physiologist, the speech therapist, the audiologist and the pathologist. How to achieve adequate selectivity of neural activation with minimal surgical invasion; how to devise biocompatible and reliable

electrodes and transmission systems and adequate spatio-temporal patterns of excitation; how optimally to encode the stimuli and yet prevent further damage to the nervous system; how to exploit what auditory clues are afforded the patient; how to assess the number and distribution of surrounding neurons—these are some of the unanswered questions (Ballantyne et al., 1978).

The fact is, however, that few groups sought to confront all these issues. Their strategies differed. For example, whereas Simmons and his Stanford colleagues made the electronics of the device a major focus for continuing research, House preferred to have development work done elsewhere (thus rapidly involving industrial contractors). Whereas some groups conducted prolonged experiments in auditory physiology (using both animals and patients), other groups had neither facilities for nor belief in the need for animal work. Because, as we shall see, the various groups differed so considerably in their research and development strategies, one cannot readily characterize the interdisciplinary nature of the development process. Different strategies entailed the recruitment and coordination of different combinations of expertise.

NEW BEGINNINGS:
COCHLEAR IMPLANTATION IN THE 1970s

Work by House, Simmons, and Michelson

In 1968, William House turned back to cochlear implants, working now with Jack Urban, the president of a small engineering firm with interests in medical electronics. In 1969 and 1970, three patients were implanted with 5-channel arrays into the cochlea introduced via the round window. Signals and power were transmitted via a transcutaneous button (a kind of small plug set into the skin behind the ear). The button was rejected in one patient at an early stage, and explantation was necessary. A second patient, deaf from advanced syphilis, moved away and work with him had to be suspended. Substantial work was done with the third patient. Despite the fact that the basial turn of cochlea only was utilized and despite the unipolar stimulation, there was evidence of pitch discrimination based on both the "place" and the "rate" of the stimulation. The work was presented at an American Otological Society conference in April 1973, and subsequently became House's first substantial publication on the subject (House and Urban, 1973). The paper discusses the various "speech coding strategies" (e.g., alternative means of presenting speech or the essentials of speech electronically) that were tried. It was after some 18 months of work on alternative strategies (which meant, in essence, different circuits and so different devices) that the patient himself chose the one he himself preferred. This turned out to be a relatively simple circuit which could be miniaturized and, for the first time, turned into a *wearable* aid. In mid-1972, the patient was allowed to take his aid home. Much of the 1973 paper is devoted to a letter from this patient describing his experiences, his progress, and his expectations.

At about this time the House group changed their strategy dramatically, and decided to concentrate their efforts on a single-channel electrode. Implantation with this began in 1972. House and his colleagues were convinced that in the current state of development multichannel implants offered no significant advantages over single-channel implants, and were very much more difficult to construct. In the five years following their switch to single-channel systems, the House group devoted a good deal of their energies to perfecting the rehabilitation offered implantees, with the objective of exploiting the limited possibilities of single-channel stimulation to the full. By October 1977, by which time 22 patients had been implanted, they had developed an extremely well-equipped otological and audiological center staffed by an otologist, audiologist, speech therapist, and psychologist. Constructing the implants, which was done outside, cost about $800. A group of British visitors was told that total patient cost was about $8,000, but this was totally funded from the private sector and no charge was made to the patient (Ballantyne et al., 1978).

While William House was moving towards a clinical procedure, Blair Simmons' approach was very different. When Stanford colleagues in electrical engineering became interested, in about 1970, the cochlear prosthesis program was reestablished. Simmons and electrical engineer Robert White applied to NIH for support for development work on a cochlear implant. Simmons' work, unlike House's, was thus subject to formal assessment by biomedical researchers and clinicians. Major doubts remained, some taking the view that the implant would necessarily damage the ear and that the benefits had not been shown to outweigh the risks. The application proved controversial. Nevertheless, in 1971 a grant was received.[2]

Quite differently from the House group, Simmons and White devoted the first years of their new investigation exclusively to developing the best possible multichannel implant, on the basis of a program of research in neurophysiology (animal experimentation) and electronics. Collaboration between otologists and electronic engineers did not prove easy. In part, according to Blair Simmons, this was because of differences in motivation. The clinicians' interest was in developing a useful device whereas he sees that of the electronic engineers as having been more in the research process: a useful source of Ph.D. projects. Every time

---

[2]Though not without difficulty. The proposal led to a site visit from a group of NIH peer reviewers, unusual (according to Simmons) for such a project. The proposal was in fact rejected by the relevant NIH study section ("on moral grounds," says Simmons, "[whereas] they're supposed to make the decision on scientific grounds"). Ultimately, however, the advice of the study section was not taken, and NIH decided to award the grant (interview with F. B. Simmons, Stanford University, April 20, 1992).

a talented graduate student completed his or her Ph.D. their expertise was lost and a new start with a new researcher had to be made (interview with B. Simmons, Stanford University, April 20, 1992).

When British observers John Ballantyne, Edward Evans, and Andrew Morrison visited Stanford in October 1977, only two (volunteer) patients had been implanted (in September), with a newly developed 4-electrode device; the objective was to "optimize stimulation strategies," although it was intended that the subjects "be provided with wearable control units in the future" (Ballantyne et al., 1978). At the time of this visit, Blair Simmons continued to regard cochlear implantation as an experimental procedure, and took the view that widespread clinical prescription of single-channel devices was premature. "All implants have been multichannel, made directly into the body of the cochlear nerve through the modiolus, in the belief that, with direct contact between electrodes and nerve fibers, thresholds would be lower, excitation would be more discrete and there would be less chance in principle of electrodes encountering 'gaps' in the array of surviving fibers than in the cochlea" (Ballantyne et al., 1978). Development work was continuing on a number of fronts. One priority was replacement of the transcutaneous button transmission system by a much more sophisticated system then undergoing tests. The British visitors were impressed by the electronic link system being developed. "This employs two separate transmission systems: an ultrasonic link transmitting pulse-coded information on when each of the four channels is active, their pulse duration, phase and amplitude; and a radio frequency link providing the power for the implanted package" (Ballantyne et al., 1978). Various aspects of the "take home" package with which patients should be supplied were still under discussion. On the basis of results from the first two patients plus one awaiting implantation it was hoped to develop "a coding system which will establish transfer of information on, say, the amplitude envelope of the acoustic signals and on the speech fundamental (laryngeal) frequencies. There is still discussion within the team about the optimal strategy which should be employed both for the psychophysical testing and for the short- and long-term attempts at coding speech signals" (Ballantyne et al., 1978).

The intention was still to keep the program small, to try to get the optimum information from small numbers of experimental subjects ("healthy English-speaking adults between 21 and 65 years of age, with total post-lingual deafness . . . adequately motivated and still functioning in society") (Ballantyne et al., 1978).

By this time Dr. Robin Michelson, an ear surgeon at the University of California, San Francisco (UCSF), who had previously worked at Stanford, had also started work. Michelson was a man of unusual background, having been trained originally as a physicist. He had also done some cat studies (which had led him to a number of theoretical conclusions that informed his subsequent clinical work[3]). Michelson moved rapidly to clinical investigation. His implant was constructed for him by an engineer at the Beckmann Instrument Company. In 1969–1970, four patients, three of whom had usable hearing in one ear and used acoustic aids, were implanted with temporary single-electrode systems (Michelson, 1971a). Results were mixed. Two patients had good pitch discrimination and could distinguish speech signals as such, whereas the other two heard only noise. It was decided to provide permanent implants to the two "successful" patients, "both of whom expressed enthusiasm for the sensations they had experienced and had a keen desire to proceed with the next step, a permanent implant." (The other two, plus a 31-year-old woman deaf since age 3 with little residual hearing, were in fact permanently implanted shortly afterwards.) Results with the two successful patients were audiologically promising, since both could distinguish a pure sine wave from a square wave of the same fundamental frequency, and both had good pitch discrimination. However, neither could actually distinguish speech. Presenting his work with all five implantees at a May 1971 conference, Michelson was obliged to conclude that "the goal of usable speech recognition through a relearning process has not been obtained to date with these patients" (Michelson, 1971b). And even if a more satisfactory audiological gloss could be put on things ("The *elements* of speech recognition, however, have been attained"; Michelson, 1971b, italics added), there remained technical problems with the device itself. The system to be implanted involved a radio link, and difficulties emerged in developing a small wearable device. The first patients could not be provided with a take-home system at the time of operation, as had been intended. In 1972 Michelson implanted his sixth patient.

Climate of Conflicting Opinions

Blair Simmons has stressed that in the 1970s the climate of opinion regarding cochlear implantation changed (see Simmons, 1985). He explains this in terms of a number of factors, including a greater willingness to collaborate on the part of engineers (provoked by shrinking research resources), and the fact that work was being done in different but cognate areas.[4] But any such change of

---

[3]The references subsequently made to the cat work include a "cochlea reflex" whereby stimulation of one ear was said to inhibit the sensitivity of the opposite ear for the same frequency (used as an indicator of hearing in a laboratory animal); destruction of the organ of Corti after long-term implantation; and the possibility of producing pitch discrimination without a multiple electrode but with a uniform electrical field within the cochlea produced by a simple bipolar electrode.

[4]"The second factor concerned blindness not hearing. Brindley's experiments in London on stimulating the human visual cortex of blind persons caused considerable excitement in the United States in the early 1970s. As we all know, blindness has considerably more emotional and political impact than deafness. NIH established an intramural program whose purpose was to investigate cortical and subcortical stimulation, both for blindness and for treatment of other neurological disorders. . . . Hearing became a major interest when it became obvious that a cortical visual implant was not going to work . . ." (Simmons, 1985).

climate came about gradually. At the beginning of the 1970s there were major differences in opinion regarding what had actually been achieved, even among those committed to the general value of implantation. A workshop that took place in San Francisco in 1974 showed disagreement about the experimental or "experimental/therapeutic" status of the technique (with most inclining to the former view); about the proven (or not) value of the single-channel implant; and about the benefit to be expected from a future multichannel device. There was nevertheless a general view that the future was rosy, that of the 300,000 profoundly deaf individuals in the United States "as many as two thirds of these patients might derive some potential benefit from an implant device" (Merzenich and Sooy, 1974). Within the basic research community, however, there was still definite opposition. Scientists working in the physiology and neurology of hearing took the view that present knowledge provided insufficient grounds for "human experimentation." Whatever clinicians' desire to "oralize" the "deaf and dumb," the basis on which to design an implant properly was simply lacking. To proceed on the basis of what was then known was professionally and ethically unacceptable.

The critical view was given particularly authoritative expression by Nelson Kiang of the Massachusetts Institute of Technology and the Massachusetts Eye and Ear Infirmary. Kiang's view at this time was that providing speech recognition through electrical stimulation was in theory feasible, though never with a single-channel implant. However, for multichannel devices to yield more satisfactory results, the electrodes would have to be positioned with considerable accuracy (a problem for the surgeon) and the output characteristics of the device would have to be properly specified. This was a problem for physiology. "If the information available at the level of the nerve is improperly coded," wrote Kiang and Moxon, "it may prove difficult, even with training, to use a prosthetic device in communication tasks" (Kiang and Moxon, 1972). Kiang stressed that, at that time, too little was known of how the central nervous system processed auditory information for prosthesis design to be based on much more than guesswork. Further animal studies were necessary before clinical work was taken further. Kiang was profoundly opposed to what a number of clinicians were doing, and made his views known in various ways. He delivered a scathing attack on the House-Urban presentation at the April 1973 American Otological Society meeting.[5] House responded simply that "I am trying to do everything I can to improve the patient's situation."

Responses to critical opinions like those set out with authority by Kiang differed. House simply soldiered on, in effect implanting single-channel devices (the first of which had been implanted in October 1972) on a (limited) clinical

---

[5]"Dr. House's results are no different from those of previous workers except that the criteria applied to the definition of success have been lowered. Enthusiastic testimonials from patients cannot take the place of objective measures of performance capabilities . . . ."

basis. Simmons had himself decided temporarily to focus on experimental studies on animals and engineering work. The UCSF group, however, changed focus, in a sense internalizing the debate that was taking place. Michael Merzenich, a physiologist, was recruited by Francis Sooy, chair of the ear-nose-throat (ENT) department. In fact, Merzenich had a joint appointment with the physiology department, and to begin with he had no desire to get involved with cochlear implantation. Indeed, he was convinced that Michelson's understanding of what the implant was to do was erroneous. Michelson's requests that he see one of the implant patients were resisted, until finally Merzenich agreed on condition that he could himself test the patient's hearing. This he did:

> I was flabbergasted. I was amazed what this person could hear and distinguish with the single channel. I knew enough about Vocoders, about speech representation, about speech processors to know that, if you could get that much information from a base channel then there was a possibility that you could represent speech. . . . I more or less instantly got the bug. I thought this was something that should be studied (interview with Michael Merzenich, Nottingham, September 1992).

Despite the universal opinion of physiologist colleagues (including his own department head) that he should not get involved with cochlear implantation, Merzenich decided to collaborate with Michelson. He devoted the years 1972–1973 principally to animal studies: partly investigations of the long-term effects of implantation and electrical stimulation on the cochlea, partly investigations aimed at understanding what kind of pattern of controlled stimulation might generate adequate speech representation. This work was to provide indications as to the design of a multichannel system. Development work proceeded cautiously, with each of a series of improved designs implanted in small numbers of patients. In 1979, and then in collaboration with Gerald Loeb from NIH, a new start was made and a design evolved that was subsequently to be industrially produced and tested in full-scale clinical trials. But that was only at the beginning of the 1980s.

Developing Interest Abroad

William House's work was beginning to attract interest among European clinicians, particularly in Austria, Germany, and France. A number of people listened with fascination to House's lecture at the 1973 International Otolaryngological Conference, which took place in Venice. One of these was C-H. Chouard who, often thinking back to what otologist Eyries had told him years before, speaks of having "dreamt constantly of an electrical system, a James Bond-style gadget, which would be able to alleviate the formidable handicap of total deafness" (Chouard, 1973). He read of Simmons' work and of that of House. He visited Los Angeles to see House operate. Aware of the need for expertise he did not possess, in April 1973 Chouard approached Patrick

MacLeod, director of the Laboratory of Sensory Neurophysiology of the Ecole Practique des Hautes Etudes (EPHE) in Paris. In May the two went to the Venice conference. Having listened to House, and to "two Americans from San Francisco who had been working mainly on animals," Chouard recalled that it was immediately clear to them that more than one electrode would have to be inserted. Chouard seems to have been clear from the start what his goal was, and what his strategy would have to be: "The sole interest of our idea was to allow us to obtain a certain understanding of language: this would be impossible to appreciate in the case of the cat." Technical problems of implant design and surgical strategy of course remained, and these were the subject of concentrated attention during the summer of 1973. MacLeod and Chouard wanted an implant in which the cochlea could be stimulated independently at different points along its length: the more the better. They settled for a design in which frequency bands would, as it were, be sampled and independently stimulated. In the autumn of 1973, Chouard carried out stimulation tests on a number of "deaf mutes" to see whether "typically speaking" (as he put it) the auditory nerve is active. By the end of the year three people had been implanted, and a note on what had been done appeared in *La Nouvelle Presse Médicale* (a general medical journal) in December 1973.

Professor Chouard was convinced by his experiences that some at least among the (totally) deaf could be made to hear by means of the implant. His strategy, like that of Dr. House, was to try to create the conditions under which cochlear implantation could be provided on a significant scale. A substantial mobilization of support was clearly needed if this was to be possible: patients, money, industrial collaboration. An effective program of rehabilitation had to be set up. This was accomplished rapidly. Dr. Claude Fugain, who was appointed to take charge of the rehabilitation, was to be a regular coauthor in years to come. The other things took longer and posed more problems. An application to DGRST (a French government agency funding research and development) was submitted early in the year. Throughout much of the year that application was pending.

In the spring of 1974, three more patients were implanted, using devices constructed by an acoustic engineer named Challier (of *Société Tout pour le Sourd* in Paris). Because the emphasis in Paris was on clinical and phonological success, rehabilitation work was vital. Implantees had to learn to make maximum use of the stimuli. Proof of success would and could only derive from *their* successful perception and production of speech. This had important implications for the overall strategy, stressed Chouard and MacLeod (1976) in *The Laryngoscope*:[6]

---

[6]The bulk of the paper is devoted, on the one hand, to discussion of factors in patient selection and, on the other, to the results obtained after rehabilitation. These are impressive: "Speech recognition

We were obliged to use experimental patients in order to test our two starting hypotheses, namely, that dividing the cochlea into electrically isolated compartments is feasible and makes speech discrimination possible. We could not use animals for this experiment, because animals, even after long conditioning, are not able to understand the human voice to such an extent as to give us enough information about the intelligibility of the received message. We could not use totally deaf patients either, because in such psychologically fragile patients no risk of failure could be assumed.

The Ninth International Congress of Audiology, which took place near Paris in May 1974, provided an important opportunity. The implantees (patients) had of course an important role to play:

> The press, the radio, the television, fond of the spectacular, make the discovery known, explaining what needs still to be done. . . . My morale is of steel. In front of the television, my patients have become "performers". . . . We make them work relentlessly, to teach them to recognize sounds, words, phrases, so that they would be able to appear before the DGRST commission which would have to grant us our subsidy (Chouard, 1973).

In April–May 1974, Chouard's work received considerable publicity in both press and television coverage, with the themes both of "deafness vanquished" and "French triumph" stressed. Though in a professional forum Chouard made clear that "we could not use totally deaf patients," the media preferred to see it otherwise. Headlines such as "HOPE for 2 million deaf and 17,000 deaf mutes"[7] or "Victory over total deafness"[8] did little to endear Chouard to his professional colleagues, however (Albinhac, 1978).

The device used in 1973–1974, with its seven separate and insulated electrodes, involved transmission via a transcutaneous Teflon plug set into the skin. This had been the source of various problems, and in a new device it would have to be replaced by some other means of transmitting power as well as an independent signal to each electrode. In the course of 1974, and with support from DGRST, Chouard found an industrial partner willing to develop and construct an improved eight-channel device. The industrial collaborator, Bertin, did not find

---

improved very quickly with training, but tone re-education was necessary. These patients must *relearn to hear*. After about a month, although the intelligibility of word lists remained poor, nearly 50 percent of a usual conversation could be understood without lip reading" (italics added).

[7]In April, 1974, *Le Parisien libéré* carried a cover story over six columns: "ESPOIR pour 2 million de sourds et 17000 sourds-muets. L'implantation d'un microstimulateur auditif peut leur rendre l'audition et la parole. C'est la révélation faite par les professeurs CHOUARD, PIALOUX et MAC-LEOD."

[8]*L'express* (May 27, 1974): "Victoire sur la surdité totale. Deux chercheurs français trouvent le moyen de guérir les sourds-muets de naissance. . . . La surdité totale est vaincue. . . . Depuis un an, en effet, quinze ex-sourds profonds parlent, entendent. Après deux mois de rééducation."

its task an easy one, and delays ensued. In late 1975, an impatient Professor Chouard was still awaiting his new device. Eventually, however, three proto-types of the Bertin eight-channel device arrived in Paris and in October and November of 1976 these prototypes were implanted.

In the new Bertin device, a high-frequency electromagnetic coupling pro-vided transmission of energy. This required an antenna attached behind the ear to a spectacles frame, and a receiver implanted in the mastoid bone. Moreover, the high-frequency modulation carried coded information to a further miniatur-ized device implanted into the skull. This decoded the messages and passed information to each of the electrodes. The total prosthesis, which was given the name "Chorimac," thus consisted of an externally worn box, an antenna, and the implanted receiver and electrodes. The external box, which weighed 2.3 kilo-grams, contained a power source which could be recharged nightly from the mains, as well as a microphone, a compressor (to keep the volume of sound within the limited dynamic range), and filters (each of which admitted sound of a different frequency band).

Consonant with his belief in the clinical utility of the technology, Chouard performed as many cochlear implants as his resources permitted: roughly one a month throughout the mid-1970s. From about 1976 he considered and then began to implant children, something which neither the House group nor any other was then doing.[9] The rate of implantation, the publicity which his work was attracting, the implantation of children: all these factors evoked some con-cern in professional (otolaryngological) circles in France,[10] though few were prepared to speak out in public against a colleague. French neurophysiologists, like their American colleagues, were also skeptical. When the question of im-planting deaf children arose, the French organization of parents of deaf children (though at that time strongly oralist) was outraged at the thought of children being used as guinea pigs in experimentation. This organization, ANPEDA, also obtained powerful expressions of dissent from leading figures in French otology, notably Professor Portmann of Bordeaux (interview with M. Portmann, Toulouse, June 1992).

Meanwhile, in London work on cochlear implantation was also beginning. Both the original impetus to try artificial stimulation and the institutional struc-ture that emerged were, however, very different from what had taken place in Paris. The ENT surgeon Ellis Douek had recently been appointed to a senior post at London's Guys Hospital, where he had been working on evoked responses.

---

[9]Ballantyne et al. comment on this: "The fact that there are apparently no problems about implant-ing juveniles and children in France means that, in time, information should become available which, at present, cannot be obtained elsewhere."

[10]A study carried out in 1978 quotes Dr. Medioni (head of the otolaryngology clinic of the Institut National des Jeunes Sourdes at Paris) as saying "No 'big name' in French otolaryngology supports Professor Chouard and his group" (Albinhac, 1978).

He had succeeded in making a significant contribution to what was becoming an area of considerable interest in the specialty. The idea that he work on artificial stimulation came from outside. The British department of health, prompted by a deafened Member of Parliament active on behalf of the disabled (Jack Ashley, now Lord Ashley), suggested to him that his specialty was doing far too little on sensorineural deafness, and why didn't he do something in that area. It was suggested that he apply to the Medical Research Council (MRC) for research support. Douek decided that, before going off to the United States and seeing what House and the others were doing, he'd try it himself. This he did, sticking an electrode to the *outside* of a patient's cochlea. Surprised by the results— which seemed to show that you could get the same kind of results House was getting with an *implanted* electrode merely by attaching an electrode to the round window—Douek went off to the MRC. Some discussion of artificial stimulation was already taking place in the MRC's Subcommittee on Sensorineural Deafness. The MRC's basic scientists were not impressed by his rudimentary experiment. Like their colleagues at NIH in Washington, MRC scientists were skeptical of the value of the approach: real language was far too complex. At this point the MRC put Douek in touch with London University phoneticist A. Fourcin:

> We went to his department, which was like a magic cavern for me, with equipment that I'd never seen, and so on. He had an apparatus, which he had invented, called a Laryngograph. He said, "Look, if we put these electrodes on someone's neck it will record the changes in the pitch of the voice. Not speech. Speech is the mouth." . . . I'd thought of speech and voice as one thing. . . . He said to me "Look at this." And there was an analysis of all the voice recordings with the Laryngograph. He said "What does that remind you of? Isn't it exactly the same pictures that you were able to produce by electrical stimulation?" (interview with E. Douek, London, May 1992).

Fourcin demonstrated to Douek how an acoustic stimulus based on voice frequencies added to the information which could be read off from the lips.

In late 1974, the MRC set up a small working group, based in a leading institute of acoustic research (the Institute of Sound and Vibration Research at Southampton University). The working group had the task of assessing existing research in the area of artificial auditory stimulation, and of recommending research to be carried out. Both Douek and Fourcin were members of this group. The working group concluded that while artificial stimulation was potentially useful "to the small number of patients who become totally deaf through a cochlear degenerative disorder," its practical achievements to date were limited (Thornton, 1977). A simple approach was recommended, involving placing a single electrode *on* the round window. Avoiding the risks of implantation, and the complex electronics of other approaches, work along these lines should yield a variety of information on pathology, physiology, psychoacoustics, and surgical techniques. The working group's recommendations, presented in 1976, were accepted by the MRC. Douek and Fourcin, together with Cambridge psychologist Moore, presented a research proposal along the lines of the working group's report, which was also accepted. In January 1977, the project, in which the Hearing Research Group at Guys Hospital (including the surgeon Douek, a medical physicist, and an audiologist), the Department of Phonetics at University College (University of London), and the Department of Experimental Psychology at Cambridge University all collaborated, started. First results were published in the course of 1977.

The project differed from others in two important respects, which were repeatedly stressed. First, deriving from Douek's initial experiment, was the view that a less invasive extracochlear approach should be used. The minimally invasive strategy was based on a quite different assessment of the risks of implantation: of infection; of irreversible damage to the cochlea; of corrosion of the electrode by cochlear fluid; of uncontrolled bone growth inside the cochlea. Intracochlear implantation would confront the surgeon with a dilemma, and might tempt him to jeopardize his patient's best interests:

> The risks associated with intra-cochlear intervention require that patients should have no useful hearing in either ear—this is a "nothing to lose" situation as it would be unreasonable to place a permanent implant in the ear of a patient who has some useful hearing in the other. Yet from the point of view of progress in this field few cases could be more useful, both to match sound perceived with electrical stimulation and to compare, say, the value of such stimulation with amplification in the other ear (Fourcin et al., 1979).

Second was Fourcin's important contribution: the idea that, at least at first, the implant should be used to supplement the information available from lip reading. The attempt to provide "hearing" was not a realistic goal, at least not at first.

> Our initial program of work was based on the expectation that the post-lingually totally deaf adult would depend on lip reading for speech communication, and be able to make use of any speech-relevant sensation by reference to an earlier memory of speech patterns (Fourcin et al., 1979).

The implication of this view was that the acoustic input to the implant should be not the whole speech signal, but rather those elements not available to the deaf lip reader (in effect, the fundamental frequency alone).

The unique composition of this team was reflected in its approach to assessing the utility of the implant. Psychoacoustic tests concerned the perceptions associated with different kinds of stimulating waveforms, as well as the discriminations potentially useful in speech communication situations. Speech perception tests included investigation of the ability to discriminate questions and statements on the basis of intonation, to locate stress in a spoken sentence, and so on. These tests, in effect, are based on a detailed understanding of the limitations of lip reading. Like Simmons, the London-Cambridge group had no intention of implanting large numbers or of offering a clinical service. They saw themselves (and indeed continue to see themselves) as a research team.

Threshold of a New Era

By the end of the 1970s, cochlear implantation was becoming a respectable topic of discussion. Gradually, it was acquiring a degree of credibility in professional otological circles. The results of an independent assessment of House implantees, which showed modest but definite benefit (Bilger et al., 1977), contributed significantly in this respect. Also in 1977, the British department of health invited a group of three experts (two ear surgeons and a neurophysiologist) to review current efforts in the area of electrical stimulation of the inner ear and to make recommendations as to what British commitment to the area should be. In October 1977, these experts visited all active U.S. centers including, as already mentioned, the House group and the Stanford group. Their report (Ballantyne et al., 1978) is in fact critical of the *overall* effort in a number of respects,[11] while nevertheless accepting the promise of the technique. Viewing full-scale clinical provision as premature, Ballantyne, Evans, and Morrison in 1978 thus recommended a cautious approach in Britain, starting with a careful evaluation of the single-channel implant.

In the period 1978–1982, however, industrial corporations were beginning to become interested. A recent analysis of the growth of industrial involvement in cochlear implants speaks of "a period of trial and negotiations between 1978 to 1982 as firms and academicians attempted to enter into licensing agreements" (Garud and van de Ven, 1989). These beginnings of an "inter-organizational field" were not easy, and a number of attempted collaborations soon foundered.[12] There is no doubt, however, that by 1982 a new era in the history of cochlear implantation had begun. Ballantyne, Evans, and Morrison bear witness to this. In 1982, these British experts published an update of their earlier report

---

[11]"There seems to have been inadequate appreciation and application of the basic physiological and psychophysical information already available, on the processing of speech sounds at peripheral levels of the auditory system, by many of those controlling the implant programs. This has meant that the expected information-carrying capabilities of single-channel stimulation (e.g., prosodic and voicing cues) have been but little exploited . . . It is surprising and extremely disappointing to note that *unequivocal* quantitative data on the benefits of cochlear implantation [compared to high-powered hearing aids and vibrotactile aids] are as yet not available . . ." .

[12]Thus in 1977 3M was approached by Graeme Clark's group at the University of Melbourne, which was interested in commercializing its cochlear implant technology. This proved abortive and Clark, with major support from the Australian government, turned elsewhere. Between 1978 and 1982 3M worked with Michelson at the University of California, San Francisco. A UCSF-3M device was developed and implanted into two or three individuals in 1980–1981. When this agreement was terminated in 1982, UCSF went elsewhere, while (in 1981) 3M entered into licensing agreements with both House and a group at the University of Vienna.

(Ballantyne et al., 1982). In it, they argue that progress in the intervening period has been such as to lead them to revise their earlier emphasis on caution. Despite continuing uncertainty as to the relative utility of single-channel and multichannel implants, the value of the technique has been proven. Ballantyne and colleagues recommended that the United Kingdom establish a limited number of implant centers forthwith, concentrating on patients with whom success is to be expected, and working according to a common protocol.

THE "CLINICIANS," THE "EXPERIMENTALISTS," AND THE ESTABLISHING OF CLINICAL FEASIBILITY

Among those otologists working on cochlear implantation William House is generally acknowledged as the "founding father." His place of honor at international conferences and the frequent demand for his recollections of the "early years" are witness to his status among his colleagues. Why should this be, given the previous history of work on electrophonic effects, and given the enormous criticism which his work received? The answer has to be sought in House's contribution to the stabilization of a clinical context for work on electrical stimulation. It was House's work, more than that of Simmons or Michelson and Merzenich, that attracted the attention of European otologists. It was House, and then in the same sort of way Chouard in France, who tried rapidly to establish a means of providing "the deaf" with an auditory prosthesis. The strategy adopted had a number of elements.

First, the claims of basic scientists that "it would not work given current knowledge" had to be countered. This was done by showing that it simply did, by "letting the patients speak." Patients were "made to speak" in various ways. One way, traditional in pathological approaches to the deaf, was simply to present live patients to an audience. A successful performance by a oralized individual is a traditional form of persuasion. Ballantyne et al. (1978) visiting House's institute, describe such a performance:

> Five implanted subjects were demonstrated to an audience which, in addition to ourselves, included visitors from Germany and the United States. They came in one at a time and sat on a platform, where they were interviewed by . . . a teacher of the deaf who is Director of Rehabilitation at the Center.

Similarly, Chouard wrote of his patients "performing" on television, while House devoted a large part of his first major article on implantation to the "testimony" of a patient. The latter's account of his successful social functioning bore witness to what had been—and thus could be—achieved. For a lay public, and indeed for many clinicians, such performances are far more convincing than any statistical analysis of word-recognition tests. Moreover, such individual experiences—with their references to the rediscovered delights of music or bird song—

are far more newsworthy than are dry statistics and complex batteries of audio-logical tests.

Second, the claims of medical colleagues that, given limited knowledge both of benefits and of possible damage, this kind of "human experimentation" was wrong had also to be countered. This could be done by arguing that it was not correct to view what was being done as "experimentation." Under attack by Kiang in 1973, as discussed earlier, House used this argument:

> I am trying to do everything I can to improve the patient's situation. That is basically different from an animal experiment in which I am required for scien-tific reasons to sacrifice the life of the animal. . . . If I put an electrode in a patient's ear, will it cause some serious harm to the patient? If not, and if there is some chance of benefiting the patient, is whatever the risk that is involved worthwhile? . . . I, therefore, think that this whole matter of human experimen-tation is not applicable in this case because we are doing everything we can for the welfare of these patients . . . (House, 1973).

Insofar as circumstances and resources permitted, both House and Chouard tried as nearly as possible actually to *offer* a clinical service from the mid-1970s. That implied considerable attention to patient recruitment (of as large numbers as possible, but also to characteristics likely to lead to success) and to rehabilitation (both House and Chouard took great pains to establish an effective rehabilitative regime, involving speech therapists, audiologists, and so on) as quickly as pos-sible. It was these colleagues whose job it ultimately was to "make the patients speak." It also implied attention at an early stage to the problem of fabricating adequate prostheses at reasonable cost. House chose to start implanting single-channel devices in 1972 because (he argued) there was no reason to suppose that they were inferior *and* because they could be fabricated much more easily at very much less cost. Chouard very rapidly sought an industrial partner (Bertin), which began to produce prostheses for his use in 1975, and was ultimately able to scale up production.

It is reasonable to interpret these efforts at creating a stable clinical context in which work on implantation could be pursued in terms of notions of "mobili-zation" or "enrollment"—of colleague otologists and audiologists, willing to re-fer possible implant candidates; of industry viewing an interesting potential mar-ket; and of health authorities willing to bear the costs of providing prostheses to selected patients. Successes and failures in this respect are highly dependent on national contingencies and political alignments. For example, Chouard began to implant children at a time when professional consensus ruled this out in other countries. Whatever the moral or scientific arguments for and against his views, it did mean that Chouard extended the kind of service he sought to provide. On the other hand, it was this decision which, by antagonizing the powerful parents' organization ANPEDA, evoked a critical response from the previously silent profession.

Most important of all, deaf or deafened individuals had to come to conceive of themselves in relation to the new technology. The category of "potential implant candidate" had to be created. To be effective, this category had to come to inform public thinking, transcending "esoteric" scientific circles. In this, the mass media were able to play a most useful role. Whatever the misrepresentation entailed in newspaper reports of "making the deaf hear," where a study may in fact have been based on implantees with considerable residual hearing, such reports probably contributed importantly to the reshaping of public perceptions.

The activities of Blair Simmons and of Ellis Douek diverge significantly from this picture. Both remained committed to implanting on a very small scale, and throughout the period with which this paper is concerned both continued to believe that the procedure had to be regarded as experimental. The significance of media "hype" for them was more subtle and more complex.

In understanding this different approach, Renée Fox's work on transplant surgeons provides a useful starting point. Fox noted that, despite their common commitment to pushing medicine beyond existing frontiers, ". . . only some of these men wield their microscopes as often as their scalpels and work with their laboratory dogs as much as with their patients" (Fox and Swazey, 1974). The "experimentalist surgeons" are "more inclined to stress the importance of caution as well as thoroughness in human transplantation and to advocate that it still be confined to a relatively limited number of well-studied patients." The distinction we need to make here is of a similar sort, although more is entailed than differences in personal orientation to innovative surgery.

Experimentally oriented otologists confronted different problems and rapidly became embedded in different patterns of collaboration from those therapeutically oriented otologists. Simmons started work again, in 1971, only when he could be sure of adequate collaboration from university colleagues in electrical engineering. At UCSF, ENT chair Sooy's early perceptiveness led to the constitution of an interdisciplinary team in which physiologist Merzenich came to play a central role. In London, Douek's early interest in implantation would soon have been frustrated if he had not made the acquaintance of the phoneticist Fourcin, who himself insisted on the need for a psychologist (Moore) in the team. The groups so constituted differ widely in structure from one another, as do their scientific priorities and ultimate clinical goals. Scientifically and clinically the London group, with their commitment to a clear strategy of implant use (the provision of "voice" as a supplement to information which could be read from the lips), as well as to an extracochlear implant, differ considerably from the others. Stressing as they do the experimental nature of implantation, these surgeons were dependent upon positive evaluation in biomedical research circles. Funding by NIH and MRC was vital for Simmons and Douek, and negative decisions could have put paid to their work. This was a quite different situation from that in which House and Chouard worked, for their work was dependent upon quite different financial sources, and upon the collaboration of audiologists and speech therapists, not physiologists and psychologists.

The "experimental" and the "clinical" approaches have not easily coexisted, and have sometimes sought to undermine each other. After all, if the technology is experimental (according to some), how convincingly can it be argued in public (by others) that "the deaf *can* be made to hear"? The "experimentalists" contested the attempts of "clinicians" (in their view premature) at forming a category of "potential implant candidates" in the public consciousness. Thus, where Michelson in his 1971 papers and House in his 1973 paper with Urban were already referring to those implanted as *patients*, Simmons continued to speak of *subjects* as late as 1979 (Simmons, 1979).[13] In a variety of ways the status of the procedure (see above) and the primacy of scientific experiment versus doing and seeing were being debated.

When, at the 1973 meeting, Nelson Kiang argued that "while it is true that preconceived ideas can sometimes obstruct progress, it cannot be reasonable to ignore basic knowledge about how a system functions in trying to design replacement parts," a representative of the Utah group (W. H. Dobelle)[14] responded:

> I think a recent remark made in my presence by "Pim" Kolff, inventor of the artificial kidney, is very important and bears repeating. When asked about the fact that, after 30 years, the artificial kidney was still not fully understood, he replied, "If I really worried how it worked, I would still be studying membrane transport in cellophane, instead of building the first artificial kidney." I feel the same way about the auditory prosthesis. If it works, I will take it. Auditory physiologists like you, Dr. Kiang, can then try to explain why (Dobelle, 1973).

Related to this is a contest over the basis of authority in the emergent field. Douek offers a clear illustration of this contest. He tells of a conference which took place in the United States, at which Dr. House asked to be the first to speak:

> And he got up and he said, "Before we present our papers I think each one of us has to say first of all how many cases he has implanted. Because that would give us a clue as to the validity of their findings." Now everybody else crumbled, because he had implanted 300 people, and everybody else had implanted 20 or something like that. But I was the second to speak. And I scotched it for ever. I got up and I said, "I think that I have to explain to you first of all what we are doing, our team in London. I have to say that we are deeply grateful to Dr. House because he has really made it possible for all of us to do the work.

---

[13]Curiously, the Fourcin paper of this same year (Fourcin et al., 1979) is actually inconsistent in this respect, using both terms at different points in the paper!

[14]W. H. Dobelle worked in the Institute for Biomedical Engineering at the University of Utah, and was himself involved in experimental studies of electrical stimulation at this time. Within this institute, and inspired by Willem Kolff, work was proceeding in parallel on a number of artificial organs and limbs.

None of us would have any funding at all if it hadn't been for the publicity with which he is surrounded. . . . This is true. . . . We are grateful. He also implants vast numbers of people. . . . We don't do that. We are a research team, and we are paid by the Medical Research Council to do research, not to treat people. . . . Now if you have come here to buy an implant, buy Dr. House's. He can sell it. . . . But what we are doing is the *research* to give you the implant of tomorrow" (interview with Ellis Douek, London, May 1992).

CONCLUSIONS

A theoretical starting point for this reconstruction of the early history of cochlear implantation was the idea, derived from earlier work, that the lack of preexisting structures of provision and of appropriate devices for the sensorineurally deaf would present innovators with special problems. My earlier work on diagnostic imaging devices (Blume, 1992) had suggested that assembling the necessary variety of skills and competences, securing agreement as to how (and among whom) the value of the new technique was to be assessed, establishing what kind of industrial expertise provided commercial advantage— all of these things would be problematic. And so they turn out to have been, but also in ways that could not have been predicted on the basis of the earlier work.

I have structured this account around the notion of "establishing clinical feasibility" because it seemed that this was the central accomplishment of the early period (and specifically of the 1970s). Those committed to the new technology were obliged to demonstrate, to the satisfaction of those concerned, that cochlear implantation seemed likely to provide benefits to the hearing-impaired. Who were "those concerned?" In the case of diagnostic imaging devices the question was rather simple, given the professional control that radiologists exercise over the production and interpretation of diagnostic images. In the present case matters are less simple, since the range of professions concerned is larger (otologists, audiologists, and speech therapists, among others). Moreover, and most important, deaf or deafened individuals also have to come to see the new device as of potential value to them. Because of this, accounts of the technology in the mass media, emphasizing the rediscovery of bird song or music or hearing the voice of one's child—however exaggerated the accounts may have been— played a vital role. "Establishing clinical feasibility" could not take place, as it did in the case of diagnostic imaging devices, in the pages of scientific and professional journals alone. That, of necessity, made it a more difficult process.

Some of those involved (including both leading members of the medical profession and leading biomedical researchers) were unhappy at this, and felt this broadening of the context of debate to have been premature and improper. The vast force of public opinion, dominated as it is by a passionate desire to see medicine vanquish deafness and all other "ills" that flesh is heir to, was all too readily mobilized. Otologists who saw cochlear implantation as a potentially valuable, but still experimental, technology had no need to recruit large numbers of implant candidates. What they needed was complex networks of scientific collaborators, to enable them to develop prostheses as safe, as effective, and as fitted to the job as was possible. Groups established along these lines not only differed profoundly from the more "therapeutic" groups but also among themselves. Combinations of expertise differed and were typically more fluid, and the relative emphasis given to different problematizations reflected scientific backgrounds. Whereas the therapeutic groups typically sought at an early stage to have a suitable device fabricated for implant, these experimental groups typically entered hesitantly and slowly into licensing agreements.

It is therefore difficult simply to characterize the interdisciplinarity of work on cochlear implantation. It was the first group—always willing to run ahead of, and even ignore, the scientific evidence—who, as it were, made the running. They it was who can be credited with securing a degree of professional support for implantation, and for attracting the interest of industry, by 1982. The field was starting to grow rapidly, so that by this time more than 200 people had been implanted (160 by House and his collaborators alone).

A few words are necessary by way of epilogue. Implicit in all the work we have discussed has been an unquestioned identification of deafness with pathology of the organ of hearing. The deaf are frequently referred to as "patients," even though few profoundly deaf adults seek medical help with their deafness. Coincidentally or not, by the early 1980s a quite different perspective on deafness was gaining credibility, largely thanks to work by linguists demonstrating the complex morphological and syntactic structures of the sign languages of the deaf (Grosjean, 1982). This work provided the basis for renewed claims on the part of the deaf to be regarded as, not a collection of hearing-impaired individuals in need of medical help, but a linguistic community. From this perspective cochlear implantation has come to be seen as a threat: exemplifying precisely the medical/pathological view of deafness that has to be opposed. It is House, who had become the hero of the story that otologists tell, who is the principal villain in this alternative rendering. The public at large, however, can more readily identify (or empathize) with House's "patients" than with Simmons' "subjects." The media, too, prefer to present technological medicine as a series of wondrous achievements, so that the "intrepid pioneer" and not his cautious critics attracts the popular following. Yet despite approvals by the U.S. Food and Drug Administration (in 1984 and in 1990), early assessments of the numbers who would seek cochlear implantation have proved to be wildly high. No one involved, in the 1970s, remotely suspected that the deaf would not come forwards in droves. No one involved had the slightest notion that the deaf could conceivably perceive their deafness in terms other than those of medicine. It is only recently that an alternative history of cochlear implantation—as a new chapter in the oppression of deaf language and culture—has begun to be written (Lane, 1992).

REFERENCES

Albinhac, D. 1978. Les implants cochleaires: Contribution à l'histoire de l'experimentation humaine. Thèse, Ecole Nationale de la Santé Publique, Rennes.

Andreef, A. M., Volokhov, A. A., and Gersuni, G. V. 1935. On the electrical excitability of the human ear. On the effect of alternating currents on the affected auditory apparatus. *Journal of Physiology USSR* 18:250.

Ballantyne, J. C., Evans, E. F., and Morrison, A. W. 1978. *Electrical Auditory Stimulation in the Management of Profound Hearing Loss*. Supplement to *Journal of Laryngology and Otology*.

Ballantyne, J. C., Evans, E. F., and Morrison, A. W. 1982. Electrical auditory stimulation in the management of profound hearing loss. *Journal of Laryngology and Otology* 96:811.

Bilger, R., Black, F., Hopkinson, N., et al. 1977. Evaluation of patients presently fitted with implanted auditory prostheses. *Annals of Otology, Rhinology, and Laryngology* 86(suppl. 38):92–140.

Blume, S. S. 1992. *Insight and Industry*. Cambridge, Mass.: MIT Press.

Bordley, J. E., and Brookhouser, P. E. 1979. The history of otology. In: L. J. Bradford and W. G. Hardy, eds. *Hearing and Hearing Impairment*. New York: Grune and Stratton.

Chouard, C-H. 1973. *Entendre sans Oreilles*. Paris: Robert Laffont.

Chouard, C-H., and MacLeod, P. 1976. Implantation of multiple electrodes for rehabilitation of total deafness: Preliminary report. *Laryngoscope* 86:1743.

Davis, H. 1935. The electrical phenomena of the cochlea and the auditory nerve. *Journal of the Acoustical Society of America* 6:205.

Djourno, A., and Eyries, C. 1957. Prosthèse auditive par excitation électrique à distance du nerf sensoriel à l'aide d'un bobinage inclus à demeure. *Presse médicale* 65:63.

Dobelle, W. H. 1973. Discussant remarks. *Annals of Otology* 82:517.

Doyle, J. B., Doyle D. H., et al. 1963. Electrical stimulation in eighth nerve deafness. *Bulletin of the Los Angeles Neurological Society* 28:148–150.

Fourcin, A. J., Rosen, S. M., Moore, B. C. J. et al. 1979. External electrical stimulation of the cochlea: Clinical, psychophysical, speech-perceptual, and histological findings. *British Journal of Audiology* 13:85.

Fox, R. C., and Swazey, J. 1974. *The Courage to Fail*. Chicago: University of Chicago Press.

Garud, R., and van de Ven, A. H. 1989. Technological innovation and industry emergence: The case of cochlear implants. In: A. H. van de Ven, H. L. Angle, and M. S. Poole, eds. *Research on the Management of Innovation: The Minnesota Studies*. New York: Harper & Row.

Grosjean, F. 1982. *Life with Two Languages: An Introduction to Bilingualism*. Cambridge, Mass.: Harvard University Press.

House, W. F. 1973. Discussant remarks. *Annals of Otology* 82:516.

House, W. F. 1985. A personal perspective on cochlear implants. In: Schindler and Merzenich, eds. *Cochlear Implants*. New York: Raven Press, p. 15.

House, W. F., and Urban, J. 1973. Long term results of electrode implantation and electronic stimulation of the cochlea in man. *Annals of Otology* 82:504.

Jones, R. C., Stevens, S. S., and Lurie, M. H. 1940. Three mechanisms of hearing by electrical stimulation. *Journal of the Acoustical Society of America* 12:281.

Jongkees, L. B. W. 1982. *Wat Bleef, Wat Verdween.* Amsterdam: University of Amsterdam.

Kiang, N. Y. S., and Moxon, E. C. 1972. Physiological considerations in artificial stimulation of the inner ear. *Annals of Otology* 81:714.

Lane, H. 1992. *The Mask of Benevolence: The Disablement of the Deaf Community in America.* New York, N.Y.: Knopf.

Lurie, M. H. 1973. Participant remarks. *Annals of Otology* 82:513.

Merzenich, M. M., and Sooy, F. A., eds. 1974. *Report on a Workshop on Cochlear Implants.* San Francisco: University of California, San Francisco.

Michelson, R. P. 1971a. Electrical stimulation of the human cochlea. *Archives of Otolaryngology* 93:317.

Michelson, R. P. 1971b. The results of electrical stimulation of the cochlea in human sensory deafness. *Annals of Otology* 80:914.

Simmons, F. B. et al. 1973. A functioning multichannel auditory nerve stimulator. A preliminary report on two human volunteers. *Acta Otolaryngologica* 87:170.

Simmons, F. B. 1985. History of cochlear implants in the United States: A personal perspective. In: Schindler and Merzenich, eds. *Cochlear Implants.* New York: Raven Press.

Simmons, F. B. et al. 1964. Electrical stimulation of the acoustic nerve and inferior colliclus in man. *Archives of Otolaryngology* 79:559.

Simmons, F. B. et al. 1965. Auditory nerve: Electrical stimulation in man. *Science* 148:104.

Simmons, F. B. 1985. History of cochlear implants in the United States: A personal perspective. In: Schindler and Merzenich, eds. *Cochlear Implants.* New York: Raven Press, p. 1.

Stevens, S. S. 1937. On hearing by electrical stimulation. *Journal of the Acoustical Society of America* 8:191.

Thornton, A. R. D., ed. 1977. *A Review of Artificial Auditory Stimulation.* Southampton, England: Institute of Sound and Vibration Research.

6

Innovation in Cardiac Imaging

STAN N. FINKELSTEIN, KEVIN NEELS, AND GREGORY K. BELL

Technological innovation has been the lifeblood of many sectors of the American economy and, as a result, managers, policymakers, and academic researchers have long sought to understand what factors encourage technological innovation and how this process can be made more productive. While innovation has been studied intensively in a wide range of contexts,[1] there remains a considerable need for a better understanding of *medical* innovation as it occurs in academic, industrial, and government research and development settings. Innovation in medical technology takes place within a unique environment that raises many complex issues regarding the need for collaboration across disciplinary lines and the moral and ethical implications of working with human subjects. Improving our understanding of this process may help us to identify points of leverage and accelerate the pace of technological innovation.

This chapter presents some preliminary findings and hypotheses drawn from field interviews with key participants who are involved in the innovation process in two important and widely used technologies that provide diagnostic information about the heart: nuclear cardiology and echocardiography. These technologies pose some especially interesting problems for innovators since, in both instances, their development and eventual successful application required col-

---

[1]Nathan Rosenberg, for example, has published a number of papers on this topic. See, for example, "The direction of technological change: Inducement mechanisms and focusing devices" (Rosenberg, 1969); "Problems in the economist's conceptualization of technological innovation" (Rosenberg, 1975); and "The influence of market demand upon innovation: A critical review of some recent empirical studies" (Rosenberg and Mowery, 1979).

laboration between individuals trained in medicine or the life sciences and those trained in engineering or the physical sciences.

Our approach has been to identify a number of distinct innovations within the overall development of each of the main technologies identified above. Through interviews with engineers, scientists, and clinicians in industry and academia who were involved in or highly knowledgeable about each development, we explored the sequences of events leading up to the innovation, the settings within which the events took place, and the backgrounds and interactions of the participants. (Several case write-ups of component innovations appear as appendixes.) Then, drawing upon the findings yielded by our research, we constructed a model to identify elements of the innovation process that seemed to be common to each of the developments we examined.

Analysis of this tentative model of the innovation process helped us to identify some points of leverage for increasing the rate and sharpening the focus of innovation. We discuss how these levers could productively stimulate changes in managerial and public policy.

Our focus upon two limited areas of technology reflects a conscious decision to opt for depth rather than breadth of analysis. With only two data points it is impossible to subject our observations and conclusions to rigorous empirical verification; thus, they should be taken as hypotheses and directions for further research rather than as firmly proven facts. Our hope is that an in-depth exploration of these two areas of innovation will provide greater insight into some of the qualitative and serendipitous aspects of the innovation process and inject some new ideas into the ongoing debate over what can and should be done to foster and support this process.

OVERVIEW OF CARDIAC IMAGING

The cardiovascular field provides an excellent opportunity to study the process of innovation. In the past 20 years especially, a number of technological advances in diagnosis and therapy have significantly changed clinical practice. Cardiology now attracts top medical school graduates and as its practice has become increasingly interventional many of these new capabilities have diffused from tertiary medical centers to the community. These developments have contributed to observed reductions in death rates from heart disease and to improvements in the quality of life.

Numerous techniques are available for producing images of the heart that provide valuable information for guiding diagnosis, patient assessment, and therapeutic intervention. From this set of techniques we have selected two areas of technology that in recent decades have seen especially significant advances: nuclear cardiology and echocardiography.[2] Nuclear medicine techniques are

---

[2]Other imaging technologies that have been used in this therapeutic area include X-ray imaging with contrast agents and magnetic resonance imaging (MRI).

TABLE 6-1   Selected Innovations in Cardiac Imaging

Echocardiography (uses ultrasound)	Nuclear Cardiology (uses radioisotope emission scintigraphy)
Two-dimensional	Thallium-201
Real time	Technetium-99 sestamibi (Tc-99 sestamibi)
Phased array	Single photon emission computerized
Pulse Doppler	tomography (SPECT)
Color flow	SPECT camera
Channel expansion (64-128)	Triple-headed camera
Transesophageal	Quantitative image interpretation
Acoustic quantification	

minimally invasive and have been used, for the most part, in patients with known or suspected coronary artery disease—the progressive blockage of the coronary arteries that can eventually lead to ischemia, angina, and heart attack. The ultrasound technique, or echocardiography, is noninvasive and has figured most prominently in the diagnosis of a variety of heart conditions other than coronary disease, such as valve disease, septal defects, and wall motion abnormalities.

As shown in Table 6-1, our study focused on successive innovations in the development of these imaging modalities. We found the two streams of innovation to be largely nonoverlapping clinically, although this may change in the future as echocardiography evolves toward a more prominent place in the evaluation of coronary artery disease patients.

Nuclear Cardiology

Although radioisotope tracer techniques have been used sporadically in cardiology since the 1920s, their use for the evaluation of myocardial blood flow and pumping ability has become widespread only within the past 15 years. With this technique, a radioisotope, given intravenously, is rapidly and selectively taken up by healthy cardiac tissue. The tracer agent emits high-energy photons whose spatial location can be detected by a scintillation camera. The pattern of high- and low-photon emission densities produces an image of the heart. The clinical utility of these images arises from the simple fact that the radioisotope is taken up only in regions of normal heart tissue with adequate blood flow. Thus, a region of scar tissue left over from a prior infarction will not take up the radioisotope and will show up on the image as a dark spot. Blockages of the coronary arteries resulting in regions of insufficient blood flow will also create dark spots.

Such an image of the heart can provide information that is unavailable through other means. One of the most important clinical applications of nuclear cardiology involves the detection and evaluation of reversible defects. In patients with coronary artery disease the adequacy of the blood flow provided by the occluded arteries depends upon the patient's level of exercise. At rest the blood flow may be adequate, thus images taken at rest may appear normal. With exercise, however, the oxygen demands of the myocardium may grow beyond what the occluded arteries can deliver, thus images taken after exercise may show defects. Such defects are characterized as reversible lesions.[3] They can be treated via therapeutic interventions such as coronary bypass surgery or angioplasty aimed at restoring normal blood flow.[4] However, defects that appear both at rest and after exercise are simply scar tissue, in contrast, a permanent defect. Such regions cannot be treated with the interventions noted above.

Nuclear cardiology techniques have found other applications in the management of coronary artery disease. Measurements taken at rest or during stress have been shown to provide important information regarding a cardiac patient's long-term prognosis. Nuclear cardiology techniques have been used extensively in patients recovering from heart attacks to determine how much myocardium and function may have been lost (Kotler and Diamond, 1990). Images taken of the blood pool during the brief period before the radioisotope is taken up by the heart can provide valuable quantitative information about the heart's pumping action.

There are at least three important categories of recent technological innovations in cardiac nuclear medicine imaging: advances in cameras and detectors; development of better isotropic labeling agents; and the wider use of computer techniques for image reconstruction and interpretation. Our research focused on five innovations within these three categories: the development of thallium-201 imaging (see Appendix A), Tc-99 sestamibi tracer (see Appendix B); the single photon emission computed tomographic (SPECT) camera; triple-headed camera; and computer-based quantitative image interpretation (see Appendix C for a review of developments in SPECT camera technology).

---

[3]The use of the term "reversible" grows out of the nature of the imaging protocol used in connection with thallium-201. This agent is administered after the patient has exercised sufficiently to raise his or her heart rate to its maximum level. The agent is then taken up by those regions of normal myocardium that have adequate blood flow. Over the next several hours, the thallium-201 redistributes to areas of normal myocardium that have blood flow at rest. The process is not unlike that which occurs when a drop of ink is released into a glass of water; over time the ink will redistribute throughout the volume of water. In the standard thallium protocol, a second image will be taken several hours after the patient has exercised. The redistribution will then have "reversed" the original lesions.

The improved imaging agent—Tc-99 sestamibi—was designed specifically to remain in those portions of the heart into which it was originally absorbed. Because it does not redistribute, its use entails a quite different protocol in which the patient receives two separate injections of the agent, each a day apart.

[4]In bypass surgery the blocked coronary arteries are surgically replaced with open vessels taken from other parts of the body. In angioplasty a catheter with a balloon on the tip is inserted into the blocked artery. Inflation of the balloon tip at the site of the blockage mechanically forces open the artery.

Echocardiography

Echocardiography employs high-frequency sound waves to generate visual images of cardiac anatomy and function. The basic principles involved are not unlike those involved in sonar. The technological basis of echocardiography fundamentally shapes the kinds of clinical information it provides. Because the nature of the signal depends strongly on the attenuation and reflection properties of the structures through which it passes, echocardiography has always had a strong anatomical focus. The high rate of image acquisition it provides has also made it a valuable tool for examining and evaluating the movement of cardiac structures.

Over the past 15 years this technology has developed substantially, and there is little evidence that the procedures now in general use exhaust its potential. In the coming years we are likely to see continuing improvements in its accuracy, the breadth of clinical information it generates, and its ease of use. And, over the long term, echocardiography may pose a substantial competitive threat to diagnostic nuclear cardiology.

The recent history of echocardiography illustrates the flexibility and power of this technology. The M-mode machines used in early clinical diagnoses could look only along a single axis, providing what was sometimes called an "ice-pick" view. An ultrasonic signal would be transmitted along this axis and reflected off any anatomical structures it encountered. As these structures moved, differences in the length of the travel path created corresponding differences in the time between emission and detection of the reflection. Originally, these machines were limited to the diagnosis of valvular disorders. A skilled clinician who could orient the machine toward a heart valve could observe how the valve moved with the beating of the heart. The later addition of scanning and more advanced signal processing capabilities enabled clinicians to generate two-dimensional images of the heart. With this development, users of echocardiography were able to examine large-scale cardiac anatomy.

The technology quickly evolved from still pictures to real-time moving images. Moving pictures provided valuable information on cardiac function. Changes in volume over the course of the beat cycle provided a basis for assessing the heart's pumping ability. By revealing wall motion abnormalities, real-time imaging also provided indirect information on the presence of scar tissue and/or ischemia.

The development of Pulse Doppler allowed echocardiography to use changes in frequency caused by the motion of the blood in the heart (i.e., the Doppler effect) to generate quantitative information about velocities. The subsequent development of Color Doppler made it possible to display this information visually through color-coding of what had previously been a gray-scale image. These capabilities made it possible for clinicians to use echocardiography to monitor the movement of blood through the heart. Using these techniques, they could detect the backwash of blood through defective heart valves or see jets of blood generated by perforations in the wall separating the right and left sides of the heart.

Other developments have increased the accuracy and usefulness of this technology. For instance, the development of reliable probes that could be inserted into the esophagus improved the resolution of these images by permitting clinicians to view the heart without the distortions caused by the passage of signals through fat, bone, and lung tissue (see Appendix D). The more recent development of acoustic quantification (AQ) using techniques to detect and monitor the boundary between the inner edge of the myocardium and the blood pool that it contains has provided automated real-time measurements of ventricular function—information that has been shown to have major prognostic significance (see Appendix E).

A number of further efforts to extend the capabilities and increase the accuracy of echocardiography are currently underway. One line of investigation aims at the development of echocardiographic contrast agents. Current efforts aim at the development of agents that generate microbubbles able to pass through the microvasculature and that would produce an ultrasonic contrast effect. If successful, these agents would make it possible to determine the amount of blood supplied to different regions of the heart—a development that would place echocardiography in direct competition with nuclear cardiology. A second line of investigation involves the development of miniature probes that can be inserted into the heart through the coronary vasculature. At least one clinician has predicted that intraluminal ultrasound imaging using these probes will eventually displace angiography as the "gold standard" for detecting and localizing coronary artery disease. A third effort is attempting to use subtle aspects of the ultrasound signal to characterize the tissues through which the signal has passed. Investigators have attempted to use this technique to identify tumors and to distinguish between scar tissue and ischemic myocardium. Successful achievement of these goals would also firmly position echocardiography as a direct competitor of nuclear cardiology.

THE INNOVATION PROCESS

To analyze and profit from the lessons our collection of case studies generated, we should first describe the innovation lifecycle, which serves as a framework for organizing and interpreting the events that have occurred during the development of these two technologies.

The innovation lifecycle consists of five distinct phases, through which most of the innovations that we studied passed. The length of a stage for a particular innovation can vary depending on the technical or clinical expertise and involvement required, scientific advances, and competitive actions. Table 6-2 is an outline of the innovation lifecycle. Evidence of its application, based upon examples drawn from our case studies, follows.

TABLE 6-2 Innovation Lifecycle

Concept	A revolutionary new product concept is often demonstrated in academia although the research may be funded by a manufacturer. The concept proves basic technological feasibility.
Prototype	The prototype is a working model of the product, not necessarily designed to resemble the actual product, but sufficient to demonstrate clinical utility and to obtain initial feedback from clinicians.
Commercialization	Production and marketing of the new product is undertaken. Much of the development effort between prototype and commercialization focuses on product design and manufacturing process issues.
Diffusion	The clinical capabilities of the product become clearer. Published articles appear rapidly as a progressively larger and more diffuse group of clinicians use the innovation.
Refinement	Evolutionary changes in the product are made to accommodate clinician requirements and to lower manufacturing costs. These changes represent incremental changes in the function and use of the innovation inspired by growing clinical and manufacturing experience.

Examples from Echocardiography and Nuclear Cardiology

Concept

An innovation in imaging typically begins with an isolated investigator demonstrating the technological feasibility of a new technique. Commonly, the investigator is operating in an academic setting and in some instances the research may be funded by an equipment manufacturer, often through the donation of equipment. Proof of feasibility typically involves the use of a jury-rig setup that is awkward to use and that produces results too crude and/or too unreliable to be useful in ordinary clinical practice. Nonetheless, these early demonstrations prove or disprove the technological feasibility of the technique. Successful demonstrations suggest that if appropriately developed the technique could be clinically useful.

Consider the Color Doppler echocardiography, tested at the University of Washington. Investigators there searching for defects in the wall separating the right and left sides of the heart and using early ultrasound equipment fed their signals into a color display that showed, through color coding, the direction of movement. Documents we reviewed state that nuclear medicine researcher David Kuhl conducted successful early work at the University of Pennsylvania on computer-assisted image reconstruction of radioisotope scans before the wide dissemination of X-ray computed tomography.[5]   In the case of nuclear cardiology's SPECT camera, the demonstration took place at the University of Michigan, where John Keyes attached an early-generation planar gamma camera to a gantry and created the "Humongatron," the first SPECT camera.

Concept development, however, need not always rely on the development of instrumentation. Initial academic work on signal attenuation at soft tissue boundaries was conducted by a bioengineer who was later hired by Hewlett-Packard (HP). His initial investigations laid the foundation for the development of prototypes to test the theories of edge detection and acoustic quantification.[6] The concept behind the development of the technetium-based sestamibi radiopharmaceutical was born from the need to create improved performance parameters. Academic investigations determined that the existing thallium imaging agent needed improvement along two specific dimensions: brightness, having to do with the number and energy levels of the emitted photons; and the distribution properties of the agent in heart tissue. Thus, the development of a prototype involved a meticulous search for an agent with the required characteristics.

Long intervals sometimes separate the proof of a concept's viability from its commercialization. Academics offered initial proof of the technological feasibility of transesophageal echocardiography (TEE) at an early date, and Diasonics, a company active in the ultrasound equipment market, developed commercial TEE probes in the early 1980s. The company ran into financial difficulties, however, and only a small number of its TEE probes were ever produced. Later, at Hewlett-Packard, an electrical engineer working with "Herman," HP's lab skeleton, was concerned about the signal attenuation problems posed by fatty tissue around the ribs as well as with the narrow window on the heart afforded by the space between the ribs. He noticed the esophagus led directly behind the heart and surmised, correctly, that it would be an ideal window through which to image the heart. When he presented the idea to clinicians they were excited and recalled the successful product Diasonics developed a few years back. In fact, a few clinicians actually had an old Diasonics probe. One could argue that the technological feasibility of the concept was proven much earlier, but the commercial success of the innovation was triggered by this engineer's rediscovery of the idea while at Hewlett-Packard.

Although, in retrospect, our study respondents seemed to be in substantial

---

[5]Tomographic imaging involves the acquisition of multiple images, typically by rotating the camera or other image acquisition device around the patient. Computer analysis of these multiple images permits the construction of a three-dimensional representation of the structure under examination. That image can then be displayed at any depth and from any angle.

Tomographic imaging stands in contrast to simpler planar or two-dimensional imaging techniques.

[6]Acoustic quantification involves the use of electrocardiographic techniques to measure the heart's pumping action in real time.

agreement about when and where these breakthroughs occurred, it was frequently noted that the eventual significance of an innovation was not usually apparent at the time of concept development. A substantial technical gulf often separated the jury-rig setup, which proved technological feasibility, from the prototype, whose performance approximated that of the final commercial system. The genuine clinical capabilities of the commercialized system are visible only in embryonic forms at the proof-of-concept phase, and considerable clinical vision and experimentation is required to unveil the innovation's full potential.

Indeed, sometimes the companies funding research conceived an application that is far removed from what eventually proved clinically useful and commercially viable. Consider the case of acoustic quantification. When Hewlett-Packard provided research funding to Washington University in St. Louis, its goal was tissue characterization—identification of ischemic heart tissue by its acoustic signature. Many did not anticipate that this research would play a significant role in the efforts to develop edge detection capabilities—that is identification of the heart/blood pool boundary—that were eventually to enable real-time measurements of ejection fraction[7] or ventricular function.

Prototype

The development of a working prototype of the imaging device or agent marks the second step in our innovation process. The capabilities of this prototype bear some resemblance to those of the unit that is eventually made available commercially. At this stage, different groups—potential users, the manufacturing experts, system designers, and so forth—have an opportunity to assess both technical and economic feasibility. Ideally, initial problems are discovered in the sketches and models and corrected, and are not incorporated into the engineering of a full-scale prototype.

Where the prototype is developed is also an important element of the innovation process. In almost all the cases we investigated, this step was carried out in an industrial setting. There was only one major exception—the development of the technetium-99 sestamibi radiopharmaceutical, which, because it did not involve development and/or operation of a complex, novel piece of equipment, could be developed by a collaborating pair of university-based research chemists at their own facilities.[8] In contrast, the development of working prototypes of ultrasound systems capable of Color Doppler flow imaging or acoustic quantifi-

---

[7]Ejection fraction is defined as the percent reduction in ventricular volume over the course of the beat cycle. A high ejection fraction (i.e., a large reduction in volume) implies strong pumping action.

[8]Although thallium-201 is also a radiopharmaceutical, its production required the use of a cyclotron, a substantial piece of equipment. Indeed, when New England Nuclear enjoyed its most commanding position within the thallium market, it began construction of the world's only privately owned linear accelerator.

cation were sizable engineering undertakings whose success required the cooperation of teams of skilled technicians. Efforts of this type are not easily organized or carried out in an academic or clinical research setting.

The prototype for HP's introduction of Color Doppler is an important example (see, also, appendix F). HP initially believed that Color Doppler would require a complete redesign of the system architecture. The existing equipment simply was not designed to accommodate so many upgrades (Color Doppler would be the eleventh in the series). Such a system redesign would require enormous time and effort; yet Color Doppler was coming on the heels of a long-overdue Pulse Doppler product and there were concerns about how long a complete redesign would take. Eventually an engineer at HP devised a prototype that allowed HP to introduce Color Doppler as a simple upgrade rather than as part of a redesigned system, thus preserving the installed-base advantage that HP was building and permitting HP to bring the product to market sooner. Even this simpler solution, however, required a sophisticated understanding of the architecture of the existing systems and input from some of HP's best engineers.

Development of a fully functional prototype is a precondition for clinical research into the properties and capabilities of the new technology. Arguably the most successful and clinically significant imaging innovations allow physicians to see things they were not able to see before. For this very reason, however, the clinical significance of such innovations may not be initially clear. Acoustic quantification is a good example. Physicians are still somewhat unsure of the clinical implications of real-time measurements of ventricular function since they have never seen such measurements before. Access to prototypes allows leading physician collaborators to explore the new technology's capabilities. Publications based on these early investigations play a significant role in defining the initial market for the new technology, facilitating its diffusion into clinical practice.

Commercialization

From prototype to commercialization, the development effort focuses on design and manufacturing issues as the sponsoring firm strives to lower costs, to improve yields, and to enhance ease of use. The goal of this effort is commercial success; relatively less attention is paid to clinical concerns beyond those identified during trials with the prototype. At the prototype stage, clinical investigators may accept a degree of unwieldiness and unreliability that would be unthinkable in a product designed to appeal to a broad market. In the process of moving to commercial-scale production, however, these aspects of the devices must be refined.

Ramping up to commercial scale for production and developing a more user-friendly interface are not simple tasks. Consider the somewhat ill-fated "Revision L," the twelfth in HP's series of echocardiography enhancements. This project involved the complete redesign of the system architecture, a task that had been postponed by the successful upgrade for Color Doppler. Much of the impetus for this project was the competitive challenge posed by Accuson, a competitor of HP in the ultrasound market. Accuson developed a 128-channel phased-array system, which was a great success in ultrasound radiology, and had plans to introduce this system to the cardiology market. There was no shared agreement among researchers at HP that 128 channels would necessarily lead to better images than the current 64-channel system. There was concern, however, that Accuson's success with a "more powerful" system in radiology would legitimize the success of 128-channel systems for echocardiography. Further, the 128-channel system was technologically challenging and offered a more appropriate platform for future expansion.

Hewlett-Packard engineers pushed ahead, but encountered two serious problems. The first was due to a change in manufacturing technology. Plans called for the use of surface mount manufacturing techniques instead of straight pin circuit board design. This new technique promised superior cost and space economies, which were achieved only after a tortuous learning period marked by extreme difficulty in debugging the new circuit boards. The second problem involved the scheduling of developmental milestones. This entire effort posed tremendous engineering challenges, not the least of which was development of an appropriate 128-channel architecture. It simply was not possible to develop all of the requisite new technologies and adhere to the project schedule. The result was cost and time overruns and lab morale problems at HP. When the system was finally introduced, several engineers and clinicians agreed that the image quality the new units yielded was no better than the 64-channel units being replaced.

Another example of the difficulties of commercializing a new technology is the development, in the early 1980s, of the multi-headed SPECT camera, which proceeded from a University of Texas laboratory to the Technicare subsidiary of Johnson & Johnson, whose engineers created a working prototype. In 1986, however, Johnson & Johnson closed down the operations of Technicare and licensed its work on the multi-headed SPECT to two start-up firms to complete the commercialization of the technology. SPECT cameras were eventually brought to market, but only after a number of different organizations had started and then abandoned the effort.

Diffusion

Diffusion of innovation is typically characterized by a process in which different categories of users become aware of and come to adopt the product. Early adopters are usually opinion leaders who learn about innovation from published scientific literature or from the marketing activities of manufacturers. Later adopters learn from earlier users with whom they are professionally and socially integrated. Some previous research on diffusion of innovation in medical equipment describes how certain kinds of product design decisions can influence how much control manufacturers exercise over innovations that flow from use by early and even later adopters (von Hippel and Finkelstein, 1979). Depending on the perceived need, manufacturers can offer a relatively open system architecture to encourage "tinkering" or a relatively closed architecture to discourage it.

As ultrasound developed for cardiac applications through the late 1970s into the 1980s, the number of expert clinical cardiologists from major academic medical centers who served as consultants to most manufacturers of the technology was relatively small. Some of those doctors provided input to manufacturers developing or offering competing products, although all the consultants insist that the confidentiality of the process was preserved. To encourage the development of new applications, manufacturers developing these early products offered relatively open architectures, which served the manufacturers' initial needs. In later-generation echocardiography products, however, manufacturers began to lose control over the publication process and the evolution of demands and expectations for the equipment.

Refinement

In the final stage of the process, feedback from users of the technology leads the manufacturer to refine the product. On the basis of clinician and manufacturer experience, evolutionary changes are made to both the product and to manufacturing process. Process improvements encompass reengineering efforts designed to lower manufacturing cost and improve yields. Product improvements are divided into two groups: those that enhance the clinician's efficiency, and those that enhance diagnostic effectiveness. Efficiency improvements to enhance ease of use are identified through observation and interviews focused on the clinician's activities. Performance parameters for efficiency must be well articulated by the clinician in order to be actionable by the engineer. For instance, a number of revisions to HP's initial imaging product were designed to make it easier to use. The system was redesigned to fit on one cart rather than two, mobility was enhanced through the addition of heavy-duty wheels and suspension systems, and the user interface was continuously updated to reduce the technical knowledge required of the clinician. In the case of transesophageal echocardiography, a number of HP's initial probes were broken because cardiologists subjected them to forces exceeding those anticipated by HP. The probe was initially designed as a transducer attached to the end of a gastroscope. Gastroenterologists are much more concerned about gentle treatment of a diseased esophagus; the cardiologist, on the other hand, just wanted a good picture and had fewer inhibitions about applying force to the probe to move it into a more favorable position.

The process of enhancing diagnostic effectiveness is far more complex than that of enhancing ease of use. In echocardiography a major part of this process was a quest for better image quality. In this field, however, image quality is a highly individualistic perception, and it proved difficult for clinicians to describe what was good or bad about an image in a way that an engineer seeking to refine the system would find meaningful. In contrast, in nuclear cardiology the short-comings of thallium-201-based images were well understood and researchers were able to develop new imaging agents and better cameras with properties designed to overcome those shortcomings. As a result, the image quality of echocardiographics improved only gradually and was not marked by the same dramatic changes found in nuclear images, especially with the introduction of the technetium isotopes.

In both fields there was also a certain degree of interplay between the development of new technological capabilities and the corresponding development of enhanced clinical insight. By their very nature, new imaging techniques tend to reveal phenomena that were not previously visible. Clinicians have to work with a new technology for a time before its implications become clear. As this occurs, it is likely to lead to further demands for system refinement.

Figure 6-1 summarizes the information collected in the case studies regarding the institutional settings within which key steps in the innovation process were carried out. A number of patterns are apparent and worthy of comment.

The most striking regularities apparent in Figure 6-1 concern the commercialization and diffusion phases of the innovation process. The former almost always took place in an industrial setting; the latter, in a clinical setting. These regularities arise almost by definition. For commercialization to occur the existence of a commercial entity is implied. Hence, by definition, commercialization takes place within industry. Similarly, diffusion is defined as the adoption of innovations by end users. Since the products that incorporate these innovations are intended for clinical use, this phase of the innovation process of necessity must take place in a clinical setting. While the resulting regularities are striking, they are, however, neither especially interesting nor unexpected.

The concept phase of the innovation process raises much more intriguing questions. At first glance, this part of the process appears highly disorderly. From innovation to innovation, different types of institutions are involved in a number of combinations, which presents a somewhat chaotic, if not serendipitous, picture. A comparison of this column to the other columns in the figure, however, does reveal one noteworthy pattern: universities are clearly much more heavily involved in this phase than in any other phase of the innovation process. The critical role of universities as a source of ideas arose repeatedly in the case studies.

A similarly noteworthy pattern is evident in the contrast between the ultrasound and nuclear cardiology prototype development phases. In the case of ultrasound, industry's role was critical and unambiguous. In nuclear cardiology,

	Concept	Prototype	Commercialization	Diffusion	Refinement
Echocardiography					
2D imaging	?	?	I	C	?
Real-time 2D	I	?	I	C	?
Phased array	U	I	I	C	?
Pulse Doppler	U C	?	I	C	?
Color Flow Doppler	U C	I	I	C	I C
128-channel	I	I	I	C	I
Transesophageal	U C	?	I	C	I C
Acoustic					
quantification	U	I	I	C	New
Nuclear Cardiology					
Thallium-201	U C G	U C G	I	C	U I C
Quantitation	U C	U C	?	C	U ? C
SPECT	U C	?	I	C	U I C
Tc-99 sestamibi	U	U	I	C	U I C
Triple-headed					
camera	U C	I	I	C	I

FIGURE 6-1 Institutional drivers of the innovation process. NOTE: U, university; I, industry; C, clinician; G, government laboratory; ?, our research to date has not allowed the elucidation of these relationships.

the contributions of the participants were much more varied. This difference seems to grow out of the nature of the technologies upon which the two fields are based: the development of working ultrasound systems was a complex undertaking requiring the cooperation of teams of engineers trained in a variety of fields ranging from materials science to signal processing. Assembling such a team is no mean feat in a university setting. In contrast, the range of technologies and system complexities that had to be mastered in nuclear cardiology were more limited and not as removed from the capabilities of university-based researchers. Even the gamma cameras used in nuclear cardiology were often constructed from commercially available computers, sensors, and other components. Thus, the nature of the technology itself often shapes the institutional environment within which innovation takes place.

In the refinement phase, in virtually all cases, contributions originated from a number of different institutional settings. Most often we see a collaboration between clinicians and industry that reflects the normal give and take between a vendor and a customer. University-based researchers also frequently participate in the process.

BARRIERS TO INNOVATION

Our interviews have enabled us to identify two potential barriers to successful innovation in medical imaging technology. The first stems from the gulf separating the engineers charged with developing imaging technology from the clinicians charged with interpreting and using the resulting images. This gulf is due, primarily, to the differences in training, knowledge, experience, and orientation that separate the two professions. A second barrier concerns changes in the environment that threaten to ossify the innovation process. For instance, new constraints governing academic research funding and clinical trials make it much more difficult to obtain a quick assessment of the potential afforded by a new technology. And the paper trail required by an expanding bureaucracy, both in the public sector and within industry, threatens to choke the innovation process.

Coste (1989), in his account of the diagnostic ultrasound market, credits a symbiotic relationship between the engineers and the clinicians as a driving force in the development of the market. Our interviews, however, offered evidence of a vast gulf separating the two parties involved in the process. While interdisciplinary research is necessary for successful innovation programs in many industries, we found the problems coordinating and combining the required clinical expertise in cardiology with required technical expertise in electrical engineering and/ or nuclear physics to be exceptionally challenging in many instances.

The differences between the players grow out of the background, culture, and language of their respective professional communities. Electrical engineers typically enter the discipline during their undergraduate education and, typically, much of their coursework is concentrated in the physical sciences. Clinical practitioners, in contrast, are more likely to have studied biological sciences as undergraduates. The practice of engineering often involves the application of well-tested formulas and rules-of-thumb. This mode of thinking is alien to physicians, who decry it as "cookbook medicine." They are taught to approach each patient as an individual, to immerse themselves in the specifics of a patient's condition, and to exercise considerable judgment in developing an individual treatment plan. Furthermore, both disciplines embrace centuries-old traditions and have developed their own languages and cultures. Until relatively recently, the two traditions have had little to do with one another.

In our case studies the industrial firms involved were heavily populated by individuals trained in engineering and/or the physical sciences. Individuals with formal clinical training were rare.[9] The clinicians, on the other hand, were generally practicing cardiologists; their knowledge of the technological possibilities of these imaging modalities was necessarily limited. Because of this disciplinary orientation, decisionmakers in the innovating firms often had only a limited appreciation of the clinical utility of the devices they were developing. Hewlett-Packard, we were told, employed electrical engineers and software designers and

---

[9]This observation applies most strongly to the early history of these organizations, and is less true now.

excelled at instrumentation; new research and development (R&D) employees were required to be capable of engineering complex electronic instruments. New England Nuclear was described as a company that was "good at making things radioactive." The company's initial commanding position in the thallium market was based on its ability to coax sustained high yields from its cyclotrons. Both companies had unique competence in engineering and the physical sciences; it just happened that the competence had profitable applications to the field of cardiac diagnostic imaging.

The clinicians, for their part, often failed to appreciate the power of the technology that would enable them to see and diagnose conditions heretofore unobserved. Until they had an opportunity to work with new images, clinicians had little basis for evaluating the utility of technological advances. Serendipity, rather than market-led demands, has often played a key role in commercial successes.

A striking dissonance between the degree of technical difficulty involved in bringing a product to market and the clinical utility that product provided was also evident in our study. Both the initial development of the phased-array ultrasound technology and HP's introduction of a 128-channel system entailed significant engineering problems and seemingly offered the clinician little in return. Neither system generated better images than the mechanical or 64-channel systems that dominated clinical practice at the time they were introduced. The development of real-time echocardiography, however, was a tremendous leap from the clinician's perspective. For the first time one could observe the beating heart without opening up a patient's chest. This clinical breakthrough posed no technological challenges of the magnitude mentioned above. And yet, the radiology ultrasound market had never before shown a need for or interest in real-time scanning capabilities. Radiologists did not examine moving objects and were not particularly concerned with motion abnormalities.

The development of Color Flow Doppler did entail the application of significant engineering expertise and has been a tremendous clinical and commercial success. Yet even this innovation had a somewhat checkered past. Pulse Doppler could convey information only on blood flow velocity; Color Flow Doppler was required to obtain information on direction and turbulence. Yet at the time HP decided to develop the product there was considerable skepticism within the medical community about its eventual clinical utility. Excitement among members of HP's engineering staff about the technology and HP's strong engineering capabilities drove the HP development process.

These observations highlight the critical role frequently played by those individuals able to bridge the gulf between the medical and engineering disciplines and cultures. Their significance is out of all proportion to their numbers.

Our investigations also confirmed an aspect of the innovation process that has long been widely recognized—one cannot simply order innovation to happen. Instead, it is necessary to create an environment that is conducive to innovation and then to stand back, in a sense, and hope for the best. In the past the network of university researchers, clinical practitioners, industrial firms, and regulatory authorities in the area of cardiac diagnostic imaging were certainly able to do this, as innovations we examined demonstrate. Many of our respondents, however, claimed the activities that make up the innovation process are harder to conduct now than they were in the past. This opinion is prevalent enough to lead us to consider whether changes in the environment have actually made it less conducive to innovation.

Respondents within industrial firms generally felt their work environment offered less room for experimentation than it had in the past. Not only did they have less time to work on personal exploratory projects, the process of acquiring materials for the construction of prototypes had become more complex and generally less flexible.

The process of clinical testing—imaging the heart of a human subject using a new device or imaging technique—seems also to have become more formal. In the early days, our respondents indicated, this process was extremely simple. Engineers who wanted to try out a new device would contact a clinician directly, and that clinician would arrange to make a patient available. It is necessary now to obtain a series of formal approvals both from the industrial firm and from the clinical institution before going near a patient. Requiring such approvals may well be a sensible step to protect patients. It does, however, raise the height of a hurdle at an important step in the innovation process.

Growing efforts by universities and university-affiliated researchers to appropriate a greater portion of the commercial value of their work might serve to slow other aspects of the innovation process in medical technology. Both our interviews and our review of the literature made it clear that collaboration between university-based researchers and industrial firms was a basic element of the innovation process (Blume, 1992). It was also clear that the nature of this interaction had changed over the period covered by our investigations, shifting from relatively open and unstructured exchanges of opinion and information to more formal arrangements involving greater compensation of university-based personnel. In the case of the new imaging agent, sestamibi, commercialization also involved the payment of substantial royalties to the Massachusetts Institute of Technology and Harvard University, where the agent was developed. Although none of our respondents identified specifically the growing commercialization of university-industry relationships as a barrier to innovation, we believe this trend bears scrutiny. It can potentially slow the exchange of ideas and information that fuels the innovation process.

Efforts to contain health care costs could slow the diffusion of new techniques into clinical practice and thereby lengthen the cycle of refinement leading to breakthroughs. Here both industrial firms and innovative clinicians are in something of a Catch-22. To the extent that a new imaging modality reveals phenomena that have never been seen before, it is almost inevitable that their clinical significance is unclear. That significance emerges only as experience with the new modality accumulates and as clinicians interpret it. However, the growing unwillingness of third-party payers to cover "experimental" procedures almost guarantees that there will be no financial support for the exploratory work involving the new modality.

It appears to us, unfortunately, that little can be done to lower many of these barriers to innovation. The combination of a stricter regulatory regime for drug and device testing with a generally more litigious environment makes it extremely unlikely that we will see a return to a less formal clinical testing environment. Financial pressures on universities and other publicly funded research institutions, such as the National Institutes of Health, suggest that we may see even greater efforts to appropriate more of the commercial value of their discoveries. And we are, of course, unlikely to see any reduction in the pressures for health care cost containment soon.

The one area in which the constraints on the innovation process can be eased is within industry itself. The challenge for an established firm like Hewlett-Packard, in echocardiography, or DuPont Merck, in nuclear cardiology, is to maintain an entrepreneurial environment in which individual visionaries have enough freedom and sufficient resources to demonstrate the value of their ideas. HP succeeded initially in meeting this challenge by setting up a small, entrepreneurial group and charging it broadly with responsibility for developing this new area of business. Unfortunately, as a company becomes bigger and better established with a broader product line and a place in the market to protect, maintenance of an appropriately entrepreneurial environment becomes difficult. Failure to do so, however, raises the risk of being overtaken by a new entrepreneurial startup company, as has occurred many times in the history of the innovations we examined.

CONCLUSION: MOVING TOWARD AN OPTIMAL R&D PROGRAM IN AN INDUSTRIAL FIRM

We conclude by offering a number of suggestions for ways to overcome these barriers and create an environment more conducive over the long term to ongoing innovations. To successfully introduce a new medical technology to the marketplace, three capabilities are required: first, access to the research community and products; second, the resources to commercialize or design, manufacture, and market the innovation; and third, clinical assessment of the technology's capacity for adequately meeting the need it was designed to fulfill. The first two requirements can be managed within a corporate research lab. The third requires access to and insights from the clinician's perspective.

The most effective tool we observed for bridging the gap between engineers and clinicians was the visionary product champion. In our case studies respondents often identified a visionary who was uniquely able to appreciate both the possibilities inherent in a technology and the clinical value of a new product embodying these new capabilities. Visionaries whose efforts were successful were essentially entrepreneurs sensing opportunities only dimly perceived by others, persuading management of the value of their ideas, and overcoming barriers to their realization. These individuals often played critically important roles in the histories of the innovations we studied. Recognizing their role and creating a supportive environment constitutes a significant step toward creation of a sustainable innovation process. Without the driving force of the engineers who developed AQ and TEE, it is doubtful that HP would have realized the potential of these innovations. And it is not clear that another firm would have supplied these products in HP's absence.

Our research provides less support for the argument that such a visionary should serve as director of the R&D department, or be in a similar position of authority. These individuals can be extraordinarily effective when given substantial amounts of authority (indeed, in some instances it seemed that the director's sheer force of personality was required to initiate and energize uncertain and stalled projects); however, a tendency of visionary product champions is to trust their own clinical and technological intuition above that of all others. They are prone to ignore ideas and suggestions emanating from other parts of the organization and other institutions. Such singleminded pursuit of an end, when espoused by the lab director, can be severely detrimental to the creativity of the other researchers so critical to the lab's productivity. Also, it is possible for a lab director to err in judging the value of a new idea, in which case, because of his position of authority, the consequences for the organization can be severe. Our fieldwork revealed instances where a visionary led an all-encompassing lab effort to introduce a breakthrough new product, only to have the product subsequently stumble, damaging the company's position of technological leadership.[10]

An alternative to leadership by a visionary is leadership by a harvester. A harvester should be an extremely accomplished technologist, but one perhaps more capable of assessing both the technical feasibility and the clinical utility of competing projects than of generating new ideas. In terms of initiating the innovation lifecycle, the role of the harvester should be to identify visionaries and charge them with project responsibilities. In the refinement stage, the harvester must constantly push the lab to anticipate and respond to clinician demands for diagnostic effectiveness for the products in the field.

The ideal lab manager would be part visionary and part harvester. The lab manager must establish guiding principles for technology development but must not become tied to the success or failure of specific projects. It is a rare indi-

---

[10]At least one respondent identified a situation in which a firm that once held a major place in a market eventually was forced to withdraw as a result of a series of poor decisions made by a strong-willed R&D director.

vidual, however, who can act both passionately and objectively while constantly evaluating the allocation of scarce R&D resources among project champions.

There are a number of other ways to integrate the clinical community more effectively into the development process for new medical technologies. One way to improve communication between clinicians and engineers is to recruit more multidisciplinary professionals such as bioengineers for the research lab. Some firms have traditionally preferred to hire the best electrical or mechanical or software engineers and encourage them to learn applications on the job. That practice reflected, in part, the culture of the workplace, but also the belief that those who would choose to be labeled as bioengineers were somehow not the most technically capable.

Clinical consultants recognized as leading practitioners in the field are an invaluable source of insight, especially regarding concept creation and image quality assessment. At least one firm we know of invites clinicians to give presentations before lab employees. These presentations provide the R&D personnel with better insights regarding coronary function, the phenomena clinicians would like to observe, and the clinical implications of information on such phenomena. As leading practitioners, these consultants may be more aware of academic work by other clinicians regarding new uses for imaging technology. Furthermore, a long-term relationship allows the consultant to acquire a greater appreciation for the capabilities of the base technology and may help generate new concepts for internal development. In both the concept and prototype stages, these practitioners represent ideal sanity checks to determine if an innovation might become the leading edge in clinical practice or be relegated to the fanatical fringe. Of course, in a highly competitive marketplace, the firm must always be aware of the security risks posed by outside consultants, especially during the prototype stage. In the early years of echocardiography the same set of clinical experts were consulted by all companies. Later, one of the companies we interviewed decided to disguise innovations before requesting clinical assessments.

The broad trends that have made clinical testing and university collaboration more formal and less flexible highlight the importance for industry of maintaining an environment conducive to innovation. The problem of an ossifying innovation process in an organization that can afford bureaucratic controls is one that arises repeatedly. The key to success is maintaining a spirit of entrepreneurship, especially important in the concept and prototype stages.[11] One of the more useful tools identified in this regard was HP's apparently unstated policy of ten percent unstructured engineering time. This "under the benches" policy seemed to be acknowledged by a majority of the original department engineers we interviewed, but most noted that such a policy was now honored more in the breach

---

[11]Paul M. Cook, CEO of Raychem Corporation, describes how his company has successfully maintained an innovative corporate culture in an interview with William Taylor (1990).

than in the observance. That 10 percent cushion, however, is said to be what permitted HP engineers to explore TEE and to propose a superior design for the upgrade of Color Flow Doppler.

Maintaining a continuing stream of medical innovations must continue to be a critical objective of the academic, industrial, clinical and governmental-based individuals who contribute to medical research and development. We hope that our work serves to stimulate additional research that will eventually accelerate the rate and alter the nature of technological change and, thus, be more responsive to society's needs.

ACKNOWLEDGMENTS

The authors gratefully acknowledge the Hewlett-Packard Company's Medical Products group for the support of this research. The views expressed are those of the authors and not of the sponsoring organization. We especially thank Ben Holmes and Larry Banks, without whose time, effort, and encouragement this work would not have been possible.

REFERENCES

Blume, S. S. 1992. *Insight and Industry: On the Dynamics of Technological Change.* Cambridge, Mass.: The MIT Press.

Coste, P. 1989. An Historical Examination of the Strategic Issues Which Influenced Technologically Entrepreneurial Firms Serving the Medical Diagnostic Ultrasound Market. Ph.D. dissertation. Claremont Graduate School.

Katz, R. 1988. *Managing Professionals in Innovative Organizations.* New York: Harper Collins.

Kotler, S. T., and G. A. Diamond. 1990. Exercise thallium-201 scintigraphy in the diagnosis and prognosis of coronary artery disease. *Annals of Internal Medicine* 113: 684–702.

Rosenberg, N. 1969. The direction of technological change: Inducement mechanisms and focusing devices. *Economic Development and Cultural Change* 18(October):1–24.

Rosenberg, N. 1975. Problems in the economist's conceptualization of technological innovation. In: *History of Political Economy*, vol. 7. Durham, N.C.: Duke University Press.

Rosenberg, N., and Mowery, D. 1979. The influence of market demand upon innovation: A critical review of some recent empirical studies. *Research Policy* 8:102–153.

von Hippel, E., and S. Finkelstein. 1979. Analysis of innovation in automated clinical chemistry analyzers. *Science and Public Policy* 6:24–37.

Taylor, W. 1990. The business of innovation: An interview with Paul Cook. *Harvard Business Review*, March–April 1990.

APPENDIX A

Thallium Imaging

The introduction and diffusion into widespread clinical practice of a workable procedure for thallium-201 cardiac perfusion imaging was based on a number of distinct discoveries and developments. The various components of the procedure currently in use were developed piecemeal by different individuals at different institutions.

One of the important preconditions for the use of thallium-201 as a perfusion imaging agent was the development of a functional gamma camera. Development of the Anger camera by Hal Anger met this need, moving camera technology beyond the plateau it had achieved in 1960s. This linked array of photomultiplier tubes permitted higher-resolution pictures of the areas of the myocardium perfused by the radioactive tracer. This basic design was substantially refined by manufacturers who increased the number of photomultiplier tubes, improved collimators, added tomographic imaging capabilities, and increased the number of scanning heads in an effort to improve resolution.

Some of the most significant early development work on the imaging agent was carried out by Elliot Leibowitz, then a radiochemist at Brookhaven National Laboratories. He described thallium as a potassium analogue and recognized the relationship between blood flow and thallium uptake by the myocardium that is the foundation of thallium's usefulness as a perfusion imaging agent. He also developed a procedure for postirradiation purification of the cyclotron-produced radioisotope that was suitable for use in commercial-scale production.

Another key step in the development of the procedure took place at Massachusetts General Hospital, where time-delayed imaging studies carried out by Jerry Pohost explored the redistribution properties of thallium-201. These studies showed that over a period of hours following the initial injection of the radioisotope, it would redistribute to those portions of the heart that had initially experienced restricted blood flow. Reversible perfusion defects, it was found, served as markers for ischemic but viable areas of the myocardium. This discovery became the foundation for the development of the exercise-rest double-imaging protocol that is still used today.

A number of regulatory factors facilitated the rapid spread of thallium imaging in clinical practice. The toxicology of thallium was well known from prior applications. In 1974, the Atomic Energy Commission announced that it was turning the regulation of radiopharmaceuticals over to the Food and Drug Administration. The actual transfer occurred 18 months later, just as the cardiac imaging procedures for thallium-201 were being refined. Thus, the FDA, because of its lack of experience, was not in a position to make onerous regulatory demands. New England Nuclear (NEN), the company leading the effort to commercialize thallium-201 for radionuclide scanning, also benefited from its location in Massachusetts, one of the so-called "agreement" states that had taken over responsibility from the federal government for the regulation of cyclotron-produced products. Thus, NEN enjoyed a somewhat simplified regulatory regime even for its nuclear operations.

By the late 1970s, numerous papers had been published documenting the diagnostic properties of thallium-201 imaging. Its value was well established as a tool for detecting the presence of coronary artery disease (CAD), for measuring the extent of viable myocardium in late-stage CAD patients, in postinfarction patients, and in patients who had undergone either angioplasty or bypass surgery. Publications appearing throughout the 1980s documented the findings of long-term follow-up studies showing that the results of thallium-201 scintigraphy were valuable in establishing prognoses for CAD patients.

As experience with thallium-201 scintigraphy accumulated, its shortcomings also became apparent. Interpretation of the images produced by the test required a fair degree of skill. Interpretations could vary from one observer to another. Constraints on camera positioning caused certain areas of the myocardium to be difficult to image—specifically, the areas served by the left circumflex artery. Patients unable to achieve maximal exercise could not be tested reliably. The energy level of the photons emitted were not ideally matched to the detection capabilities of the available gamma cameras. Thallium-201's relatively long half-life, coupled with constraints on the total amount of radiation to which a patient could be subjected, limited the dose that could be administered to a patient, which placed a ceiling on the total number of photons emitted during a test and, thus, on the absolute information content of the test. And although the redistribution properties of thallium were valuable in distinguishing between scar tissue and areas of ischemia, they also placed constraints on the testing protocol. Initial imaging had to follow injection within a limited time period or redistribution would render the test results invalid.

In the years following the widespread adoption of thallium-201 scintigraphy, efforts were made to overcome the limitations of the original testing protocol. These efforts, in turn, spawned a series of subsequent innovations. Attempts to make the interpretation process more consistent and more readily available to smaller centers led to the development of quantitative image interpretation software. Efforts to improve the ability of the test to detect perfusion defects in hard-to-image portions of cardiac anatomy lead to the development of Single Photon Emission Computerized Tomography (SPECT). Concern over failure of patients to achieve maximal stress and the effects of this failure on the test accuracy led to the use of pharmacological stress agents. Concerns over the emission profile and half-life of thallium-201 led to a search for an imaging agent based on the technetium-99 isotope. Investigators working in this area also hoped to develop an agent with more favorable redistribution properties. Their efforts led eventually to the development of Tc-99 sestamibi.

Use of thallium-201 scintigraphy has been constrained by the widespread availability of a number of competing testing modalities. The presence of coronary artery disease is often apparent simply from a patient's history and presenting symptoms. An electrocardiogram with stress testing can detect the presence of ischemia at a lower cost than thallium scintigraphy (although with less accuracy). At the other end of the spectrum, angiography is both more expensive and more invasive than thallium scintigraphy, but provides what many cardiologists regard to be superior diagnostic information. Angiography is also thought to be a prerequisite for either angioplasty or bypass surgery aimed at elimination of the underlying causes of ischemia, providing, as it does, a "road map" for the surgeon or catheterization expert.

The proper place for thallium-201 scintigraphy in this crowded field of alternatives has been the subject of sometimes spirited debate. Some have argued that the incremental information content of a thallium test, given that the patient has already undergone a stress electrocardiogram, is small and of little value. A number of investigators have attempted to identify specific subsets of patients for whom thallium test results can play a critical role in defining the course of treatment. However, despite these systematic efforts to identify the appropriate role for thallium testing, the choice of diagnostic tests continues to be strongly influenced by individual physician preferences.

APPENDIX B

Tc-99 Sestamibi Tracer

Tc-99 sestamibi is a technetium-based synthetic radioisotope with certain properties that enable it to produce images of the heart allowing for an assessment of the "viability" of cardiac muscle and the identification of the possible presence of coronary artery disease. It is regarded by many as an incremental innovation over the use of thallium as the agent for stress imaging studies.

Observations about the clinical value of technetium-99 (Tc-99) were first made in the late 1950s by Powell Richardson, a nuclear medicine physician doing research at Brookhaven National Laboratory. He used a molybdenum generator to produce substantial amounts of this agent with high isotopic purity. His work was published but his process was not patented.

The later development of the gamma camera, first by Hal Anger at the Lawrence Radiation Laboratory, stimulated this line of investigation, as well as the field of nuclear medicine as a whole. Various commercial firms, including New England Nuclear (NEN), went into the business of producing radioisotopes for medical application. One of the early products was a Tc-based agent to image bones. Thallium-201, produced by cyclotron, became the isotope of choice for cardiac imaging work.

As thallium-201 gained acceptance and the performance of stress myocardial imaging became an important part of the evaluation of patients for coronary artery disease, many sought to improve on thallium's properties. First, thallium's rapid redistribution made the nature and quality of the image highly dependent on the elapse of time following injection. Second, the cyclotron-based production process for thallium limits its accessibility.[12] Third, the relatively long half-life of thallium-201 limited the dose that could be administered to a patient. Finally, the energy profile of thallium's gamma emissions poorly fit the detection capabilities of the available cameras.

Two firms, NEN and Squibb, were known to be actively pursuing work on a Tc-99 agent for cardiac imaging in the early 1980s. NEN funded or collaborated with Deutsch at the University of Cincinnati to produce an agent in 1982. Its chemical structure was technetium dimethyl phosphene, and it was given the name "Cardiolyte." This agent was quite successful in animal studies, but when tested in humans at the Massachusetts General Hospital, it did not successfully image the human heart.

Since 1980, Alan Davison, an inorganic chemist at the Massachusetts Institute of Technology, and Alun Jones, a nuclear chemist at Harvard, had been actively pursuing research on a synthetic Tc-99 agent that would correct some of thallium's shortcomings to image the heart. They had personal relationships with staff at NEN and were working with the expectation that NEN would be interested in licensing their agent when their product was developed.

The acquisition of NEN by DuPont led to a shift in NEN's research priorities. Under DuPont's management, staff began to screen a large number of liquids for desirable properties in a search for an imaging agent of their own. Their initial lack of interest in Davison and Jones's agent can be seen as an example of the "not invented here" syndrome. DuPont eventually licensed the Davison/Jones agent—Tc-99 sestamibi—and sought FDA marketing approval. DuPont's inexperience with FDA submissions delayed the approval process by two years. Tc-99 sestamibi was approved and introduced to market in 1991, however, and by 1992 had achieved worldwide sales of over $100 million.

The Tc-99 agent eventually introduced by Squibb for cardiac imaging has not been quite as successful. Its extremely rapid washout properties make perfusion imaging even more technically challenging than with thallium-201. It has been said, however, that in the hands of a skilled operator these properties permit high patient throughput.

Clinicians have received these Tc-99 agents favorably and have adopted them for use in cardiac imaging. With regard to substituting for thallium, there is still debate over whether these new agents produce significantly more clinical information than their predecessors.

---

[12]This process required that thallium-201 be produced at a small number of cyclotron sites, from which it would be shipped to physicians. During shipment the isotope would decay. Producers overfilled vials to guarantee that enough isotope would remain viable upon arrival to permit testing, which drove up costs. It was impossible to store thallium on-site, either at the cyclotron facility or at hospitals.

APPENDIX C

Single Photon Emission Computed Tomography

The early development of Single Photon Emission Computed Tomographic (SPECT) imaging took place between 1958 and the early 1970s at the University of Pennsylvania. Dr. David Kuhl, a physician trained in nuclear medicine, and his collaborators constructed an array of radiation detectors. They were then able to produce a map of radionuclide concentration by taking sequential images of a series of cross-sectional slices. These sequential images were then available for back projection and image reconstruction and could yield information on previously unobservable physiological changes in the body. The original work was driven by the clinical need to image the brain—cardiac imaging came later.

Much of Kuhl's work preceded the development and availability of X-ray computed technology (CT) in the early 1970s, when the use of image reconstruction algorithms became commonplace. Broader application of the early SPECT research and further progress was, however, facilitated by and stimulated by the acceptance of X-ray CT.

From 1970 to 1974, Dr. John Keyes, working at the University of Michigan and the University of Rochester, adapted a gamma camera to perform cross-sectional imaging of the brain using back projection. In 1974, he and his colleagues built a rotating gamma camera, facetiously referred to as the "Humongatron," used for early brain imaging by SPECT through 1976.

Initial images produced by Keyes's camera or Kuhl's detector array were crude and needed a great deal of improvement. For instance, the term "error" was used to refer to the (qualitative) difference between the image and the actual clinical condition, but "error" encompasses several dimensions that were either actually or potentially measurable or quantifiable. These include resolution, attenuation, scatter, artifact, collimator error, and uniformity.

Three streams of innovations (independently) pursued led to image improvement. These involved improved image reconstruction algorithms, better imaging agents, and the camera itself. Development of better algorithms took place in industry and academia, but most prominently at Lawrence Berkeley Laboratory under the direction of Thomas Budinger. Published articles (1978–1980) document his contribution to the physics and mathematics of SPECT image improvement.

The wide use of SPECT for brain imaging came about only with the availability of the Tc-based imaging agents. Cardiac imaging with SPECT began to be performed in the early 1980s with thallium. Many investigators were not satisfied that the quality of the images produced by thallium-SPECT was significantly better than those taken with planar cameras. Even so, commercial SPECT systems capable of imaging the heart began to become available from a number of manufacturers between 1980 and 1983.

Around 1981, Dr. James Willerson, a cardiologist at the University of Texas at Dallas, received a grant to seed the development of a multi-headed SPECT camera. Willerson eventually forged a relationship with the Technicare (instruments) division of Johnson & Johnson to build a prototype of the new kind of camera. Clinical testing of the prototype was to begin around 1986, but was delayed for several years due to Johnson & Johnson's closure of Technicare in that year. The work was continued at two companies licensed by Johnson & Johnson, Ohio Imaging and Trionics. Ohio Imaging was later acquired by Picker. The University of Texas cardiology group finally acquired their three-headed SPECT camera from Picker in 1988. That company and several others now offer commercially available three-headed SPECT cameras.

The three-headed SPECT cameras are capable of resolution to about 7-8 mm, compared to the 20-mm resolution of the very early SPECT cameras. Clinical users, including some who had been skeptical of any improvement in accuracy with single-headed SPECT, have been more impressed with the images that are produced by these multi-detector cameras. And new cardiac imaging agents such as Tc-99 sestamibi are said to produce further improvements in the quality of SPECT images over those generated with thallium.

APPENDIX D

Transesophageal Echocardiography

Transesophageal echocardiography (TEE) uses the esophagus as a window to image the heart. An ultrasonic transducer is mounted near the tip of a modified gastroscope, which is manually inserted down the patient's throat. Controls then permit the operator to position the transducer optimally.

TEE is used in both outpatient and operating room (OR) settings. In the outpatient market TEE is ideal for imaging otherwise "difficult" patients. Obesity, large chests, and narrow spacing between the ribs all make traditional echocardiography difficult and reduce its accuracy. With TEE, the transducer can be placed close to the heart with little attenuation of the ultrasound signal due to air-filled lungs or bony structures.

In the OR setting, TEE allows the anesthesiologist to constantly monitor cardiac function once the chest cavity has been opened. The clear image it provides makes it relatively easy to detect the wall motion abnormalities that mark ischemia. Before TEE there was no other way to image cardiac function during such surgical procedures.

Although TEE represents an advance in transducer technology and remote positioning, the TEE probe was actually developed as an add-on to established echocardiography systems.

TEE began in the academic environment. In 1976, researchers mounted a transducer on a coaxial cable and used the esophagus to image the left atrium and mitral valve. In 1982, academicians brought the idea to Diasonics, which initially commercialized the product. Diasonics sold approximately 50 TEE probes, but did not pursue the market opportunity.

In 1985 an engineer at Hewlett-Packard (HP) was working with "Herman," the lab skeleton, and considering the problem of signal attenuation due to tissue around the ribs. He noticed the esophagus behind the heart and had an idea of mounting a transducer at the end of a gastroscope. When he approached clinicians with this observation they expressed considerable interest and produced for his examination a number of the old Diasonics probes.

At the time, HP was heavily involved in development of Color Flow Doppler imaging. As a result, there were few resources to spare to pursue the TEE opportunity. For the next year the engineer shepherded his underground project through the development process. Once out on the market, design deficiencies surfaced that had resulted from a poor appreciation for exactly how the device would actually be used. For instance, the engineer had talked to a number of gastroenterologists who were very concerned with the probe's potential to damage a diseased esophagus. Cardiologists, however, simply wanted to use the probe to obtain good pictures; they were not shy about applying force to the probe to position it correctly. Consequently, a number of the initial probes broke because the forces the cardiologist subjected them to were quite different from those that the engineer anticipated.

Eventually the bugs were worked out of the design, and the TEE probe became a small but significant addition to HP's electrocardiographic product line.

APPENDIX E

Acoustic Quantification

Acoustic quantification (AQ) is a technology that makes use of recognizable differences in patterns of ultrasonic back scatter to identify the "edge" of the heart, or the interface between the cardiac musculature and the blood. This software- and hardware-embodied innovation permits measurement of ventricular function on a beat-to-beat basis.

The AQ technology emerged from research conducted largely by academic engineers and physicians aimed at use of ultrasound for the characterization of tissues (i.e., for a "noninvasive biopsy"). AQ represented a successful tangent to a main line of research that had been ongoing for nearly two decades without leading to meaningful products.

Pete Melton, an academic researcher with B.S. and M.S. degrees in electrical engineering, a Ph.D. in biomedical engineering, and some experience running a large teaching hospital's clinical laboratory, began AQ work in 1978, examining the characteristics of the ultrasonic signal coming back from various tissues, especially the heart. In 1981, he and a collaborator, working at the University of Iowa, documented the differences in back scatter from the heart compared to other tissues. They published an article in 1983 showing real-time images and proposed an algorithm for identifying the edge of the heart and measuring left ventricular volume.

Melton left academia in 1984 and went to industry. After spending nine months at Diasonics, he came to the Hewlett-Packard (HP) Imaging Systems Division where he pursued this work until 1988. At HP, his assignment was to pursue tissue characterization (TC) rather than AQ. The common pathway to achieve successes in both TC and AQ diverged and the bioengineer made informal arrangements to continue his AQ work, making prototypes "quietly." To do so, he had help from two "unassigned" engineers, one specializing in hardware and one in software.

Melton did much of his work "outside the system." Clinical trials were done rather informally in collaboration with an anesthesiologist at the University of California, San Francisco, and cardiologists at Washington University (St. Louis) and the University of Iowa. Melton's work eventually led to the development of a prototype suitable for demonstration before clinicians. Their enthusiastic response convinced HP to "give the effort a project number" and initiate a full-scale development effort.

HP introduced AQ as an enhancement to its high-end cardiac ultrasound units. The company's eventual decision to emphasize AQ rather than TC was heavily influenced by the enthusiastic response of clinicians to Melton's prototype. AQ has, so far, been received quite favorably in the marketplace. HP believes it is gaining market share or at least solidifying its position as market leader because of it. Competitors acknowledge that their own products have suffered in comparison. Clinical specialists, intrigued by the AQ technology, say its real significance has yet to be established and it is still too early to say whether it will facilitate the making of noninvasive "statements" about cardiac function.

APPENDIX F

Color Flow

Doppler uses ultrasound to measure blood velocity. Initially, Doppler units were simply glorified stethoscopes—they were blind in terms of the area where blood velocity was being measured. Ideally, the clinician wanted to place a cursor on the screen and detect blood velocity at a certain point. Color flow was essentially two-dimensional Doppler allowing the clinician to measure blood flow velocity, volume, and direction. The great advantage of this technique is that it allows clinicians to detect eddies and backflow, which were evidence of abnormalities that could not be detected otherwise.

Color Flow Doppler required engineering advances in signal processing. A major issue was simply separating the imaging signal from the Doppler signal.

Engineers at Hewlett-Packard, Paul Magnin in particular, thought it was fairly obvious that physicians would like to measure and display velocity at every point in the image. They just did not know how to achieve it. After struggling to get the Doppler unit out, Magnin started to investigate color flow, developing some computer algorithms to process the signal. At the same time a paper published by the American Institute of Ultrasound Medicine from Aloka Research Labs showed an actual picture of a mechanically swept color flow image. Clearly it could be done, and done commercially. Consequently, development efforts were stepped up and from eight different algorithms, two were selected that seemed most likely to answer the call. It was not entirely clear which one would be more appropriate, so simulations were set up to test one algorithm against the other. Once clinicians saw the video of the various algorithms, however, it was not clear that color flow would be of clinical significance. Nonetheless, Hewlett-Packard pushed ahead with its development because it believed the technology has potential.

The path from concept to prototype was arduous. It seemed that color flow would require a redesign of the system architecture, which had not been designed to be upgradable. Once a redesign was begun it was nearly impossible to prevent everyone's pet projects from being added to the revision. Introduction of the product seemed to be far away. Another engineer, again working off the critical path, found a solution to move the product into the marketplace more quickly— sell it as an upgrade. Although this solution was very well received, the decision to offer Color Flow Doppler as an upgrade postponed some of the redesign problems to the next revision.

PART III

Biotechnology Innovation

7

Incentives and Focus in University and Industrial Research: The Case of Synthetic Insulin

SCOTT STERN

Within biotechnological research, university departments and firms are often organized as complementary inputs into research activities. The degree of complementarity is somewhat surprising (Arora and Gambardella, 1989), given the competition that exists between university departments and between firms. University molecular biology labs (or biologists) view each other as competitors for scarce funding and academic prestige, while similarly sized firms compete through markets and the development of appropriable products or processes. Why, then, do biotechnology firms and universities regard each other as complements, and is this relationship the result of the particular historical sequence that marked the early days of biotechnology?

This question will be attacked through a case study of insulin research in the late 1970s, an intense period which utilized and expanded upon the emerging techniques of genetic engineering. Observed interdisciplinary and interinstitutional research links will be examined to shed light upon the heterogeneous set of goals and trade-offs facing different researchers, the relative success of researchers in meeting these goals, and the effect of the research outcomes on future patterns of university-industry interaction. To provide focus, the research that is examined is centered around the expression of human insulin in *E. coli* bacteria.[1]

---

[1] In contrast to many other innovation studies, there are detailed accounts of the early years of recombinant deoxyribonucleic acid engineering, in both academic and popular publications. In particular, there is a well-written popular account of the insulin research (Hall, 1988). Further, the insulin research was widely reported contemporarily, most notably in *Science*, *Nature*, and *Cell*.

Research teams at Harvard University, the University of California at San Francisco (UCSF), and the City of Hope National Medical Center all played key roles in the development of the techniques, substances, and concepts utilized. However, Genentech, a small start-up biotechnology firm with no income and limited resources, was the organization first able to synthesize and patent human insulin, resulting in a royalty agreement with Eli Lilly. This paper contends that Genentech's *commercial* success can be understood through contrasting and comparing its goals with those of university departments, such as Harvard or UCSF.

While many authors have characterized the insulin research as a "race"—where researchers are solely focused on appropriating the commercial benefits of gene expression[2]—a great deal of insight is gained by analyzing the heterogeneity of these groups, the different strategies they pursued, and the *divergence* of their goals. Further, the insulin research, which resulted in the first significant commercial application of recombinant deoxyribonucleic acid (rDNA), conditioned the future organization of university-industry interaction. Genentech's success, often cited as a catalyst to investment in biotechnology, had the additional consequence of providing a framework for complementary university-industry interaction.

The insulin research was effective in demonstrating the relative strengths and weaknesses of firms and universities. In a nutshell, firms face strong incentives to produce products or processes in a minimum-cost manner. To achieve this goal, small start-up firms attempt to focus their efforts on a small number of projects. If these projects are unsuccessful, the firm will go bankrupt. Conversely, successful projects result in financial benefits to the scientists and investors in the corporation. In contrast, the mission of a university department or researcher is not so neatly characterized. At the very least, senior university researchers attempt to achieve three distinct goals: the training of graduate students and postdoctoral fellows, the resolution and explication of discipline-specific research inquiries, and the production of information that will be appropriable by the lab and the university. These three goals compete for priority. In other words, university researchers face trade-offs between devoting resources towards a project with potential commercial applications and devoting those resources towards the training of students and the development of experiments that will answer general scientific questions. Commercial firms do not face these trade-offs. This straightforward difference sheds light on the particular pattern of research relationships observed within this case study and, more consequentially, helps explain the success or failure of these research relationships.

The paper is organized as follows. The first three sections summarize the

---

[2]Gene expression refers to the intracellular production of a particular sequence of amino acids, which are joined into proteins such as insulin. The sequence is determined by the deoxyribonucleic acid sequence of the gene.

research under study by examining (1) the context out of which recombinant DNA techniques emerged, (2) the cast of characters who made up the primary research teams working on the insulin project, and (3) the timetable of the actual research. The next two sections detail the interdisciplinary and interinstitutional links observed within the frame of the study. These sections provide the background for the analysis and conclusions of the study, which examine the incentives of institutions and individuals in establishing and maintaining particular relationships, the cluster of characteristics that are present in the most successful of these relationships, and the effect of the insulin research on future university-industry interaction.

THE EMERGENCE OF GENETIC ENGINEERING

The insulin research is best understood in the context of the development of molecular biology and related disciplines. In the 1970s, critical advances in the techniques, instrumentation, and theory of molecular biology expanded the power and scope of DNA research, revolutionizing the practice of molecular genetics. Molecular biology, previously a prestigious basic science, was fundamentally transformed along with a host of allied disciplines. New avenues of research were opened, some with potential commercial application.

The proposal of a double helix structure for DNA by Watson and Crick in 1953,[3] the most public achievement of molecular biology, ensured the place of molecular biology as an elite science. Subsequent to Watson and Crick's work, a diverse group of researchers resolved empirical and theoretical questions concerning the function and structure of genetic material. Activation and repression of protein production, the intergenerational transmission of genetic instructions, and the relationship between the sequence of genetic information and the production of amino acids presented fundamental but manageable puzzles to researchers.

Before 1970, most of the important advances within molecular genetics were the result of studying prokaryotic (lower) organisms. Conversely, important questions within prokaryotic biology could be resolved through the use of molecular genetics. Particular research avenues within bacteriology, the study of phage,[4] for example, utilized molecular genetics to advance understanding of bacteriology as well as more general genetic phenomena. While molecular biology stood at the heart of these advances, it can be argued that the rapid pace and

---

[3]The classic popular reference concerning the discovery of the structure of DNA is James Watson's *The Double Helix* (1968), where Watson describes the intensity of the academic competition in the pursuit of the genetic structure. See also the classic textbook *Molecular Biology of the Gene* (Watson, 1976).

[4]Bacteriophage are an especially studiable type of virus which can attack bacteria. Many of the early advances in recombinant DNA occurred within the context of the study of bacteriophage.

surprising direction of discovery led to fundamental ambiguities concerning the scope of molecular biology in relation to other disciplines. Bacteriologists, organic chemists, geneticists, and classical biochemists[5] all contributed to the growing body of tools, techniques, and theory. Paul Berg, one of the most innovative researchers within the field and a biochemist by training, argues that molecular biologists were united by similar beliefs about the proper level at which to understand cell behavior: "Someone who would have called themselves a molecular biologist . . . would want to understand the phenomena at the molecular level" (telephone interview with Paul Berg, Professor of Biochemistry, Stanford University, February 17, 1993). This approach necessitated asking questions of a more fundamental nature than those asked within much of the mainstream of classical biochemistry. While perhaps providing the advantage of analytical depth and rigor, pre-1970s molecular biology suffered from tools that were inadequate for seriously studying eukaryotic (higher) organisms. Thus, the whole of biochemistry, much of it focused on "the characterization of metabolic pathways . . . of the more numerous and immediately useful proteins" (Kenney, 1986, p. 12), was affected but not transformed by molecular genetics. This distinction held as long as understanding of the physiological events of eukaryotes could not be greatly enhanced through the use of molecular genetic approaches.

After 1970, critical advances in technique, instrumentation, and theory overcame many of the barriers that had slowed the adoption of molecular genetics. The most public and startling of these advances was the gene-splicing technique pioneered by Stanley Cohen and Herbert Boyer in 1973. Along with work by Jackson, Symons, and Berg, the potential to manipulate—to change—the genetic code and subsequent protein production of an organism became feasible through use of restriction enzymes[7] developed by Boyer (Johnson, 1983). This technique "has allowed for the first time the analysis of individual eukaryotic genes as well as the study of the organization of genetic information in higher organisms," as well as "enabled modification of the genetic makeup of bacteria and unicellular eukaryotic organisms so as to render them capable of producing gene products encoded by the DNA of higher eukaryotes" (Cohen, 1982, p. 21). The Cohen-Boyer technique had a broad effect on biology and biochemistry. Not only did it aid in the resolution of long-standing questions, it opened up the possibility of asking fundamentally new questions. Not surprisingly, the fundamental novelty of the technique led to serious questions of ethics and safety. Perhaps a bit more

---

[5]The definition and boundaries of each of these disciplines have changed over time, but the textbook definition or the relative scope of each has not changed nearly as much as that of molecular biology.

[6]Restriction enzymes are the critical material in "cutting" up genetic material for the purpose of extracting specific DNA strands. These strands are then spliced into plasmids for the purpose of insertion into bacteria.

surprising, heated debate among molecular biologists resulted in a self-imposed two-year moratorium on recombinant DNA research.[7]

While recombinant DNA experimentation was halted, complementary techniques for DNA sequencing, gene synthesis, and gene detection advanced considerably. DNA sequencing yields the order of the nucleotides (A, C, T, or G)[8] along a strand of DNA. This information is sufficient to predict the amino acids and proteins that can be produced by an organism. DNA sequencing methods were advanced through refinement of *gel electrophoresis*.[9] The most important advances were simultaneously pioneered by Walter Gilbert[10] and Allan Maxam at Harvard University and A. R. Coulson and Frederick Sanger at Cambridge University. Their primary achievement was "the separation of DNA molecules that differ in length by only one nucleotide" (Kolata, 1976, p. 645). The sequencing techniques developed at Harvard and Cambridge were reported to "herald a new era in molecular biology—an era in which . . . long-standing problems of DNA structure, sequence, organization and function will become clear" (Kolata, 1976, p. 647). The Gilbert-Maxam technique effectively reduced sequencing time by an order of magnitude. Moreover, sequencing was (and is) one of the most time-consuming activities of the molecular biologist. It is a useful measure of the technique's utility to note that while Herbert Boyer and Stanley Cohen have not received the Nobel Prize for their gene-splicing technique, Gilbert and Sanger shared the 1980 Nobel Prize in Chemistry for the sequencing advances.

Artificial gene synthesis was also pioneered during the moratorium on rDNA research. Har Gobind Khorana, of the Massachusetts Institute of Technology, fabricated an artificial gene by stringing together nucleotides in the appropriate order.[11] The synthetic technique, requiring "9 years of work by 24 postdoctoral fellows," was "hailed . . . as a major accomplishment in genetics" (Maugh, 1976). Khorana's work was considered an excellent piece of basic research, whereby

---

[7]An excellent review of this debate and details of the regulation has been performed by Krimsky (1982). While the rDNA controversy will not be reviewed here, the role of regulation in the insulin research is examined. The chief regulator of rDNA experimentation in the late 1970s was the Recombinant DNA Advisory Committee (RAC), which operated under the auspices of the National Institutes of Health. The most important component of regulation was the issuance of standards of safety care for different classes of experiments. P1, the most lax standard, required little adjustment from standard laboratory procedure. P4, the strictest standard, was reserved for experiments with dangerous or human genetic material and could only be performed in the equivalent of a military biowarfare lab.

[8]Adenine, cytosine, thymine, and guanine, respectively.

[9]*Gel electrophoresis* involves the separation and identification of molecules in gels. Separation is achieved through the application of an electric field upon ion molecules in an electrolyte solution. Differential rates of migration of the ion molecules allow for identification (Braithwaite and Smith, 1985, p. 70).

[10]Gilbert is one of the lab chiefs within this case study of insulin. The insulin research was a particular application of the overall research direction of Gilbert's lab after the sequencing breakthrough.

[11]The base elements of DNA can be obtained commercially rather inexpensively.

"the goal is to learn more about the gene itself and how it is regulated" (Maugh, 1976). However, the commercial application of the technique was also noted: "One suggestion is to incorporate a gene for insulin in a bacteria such as *E. coli* so that the valuable protein could be harvested from bacterial fermentation instead of from animals" (Maugh, 1976). As will be seen, Genentech pursued *exactly* this strategy.

Innovations in gene splicing, DNA sequencing, and gene synthesis required advances in both technique and instrumentation.[12] Further, molecular genetic theory was informed, indeed transformed, by the expanded range of manipulation and observation of genetic material. With the issuance of National Institutes of Health (NIH) regulations in June 1976, rDNA experimentation resumed. Research proceeded at an extraordinary pace. However, it is the direction of some of this research, rather than its pace, which is of primary concern here. An influential group of researchers perceived the opportunity to *apply* the new techniques. Labs exploring gene expression with rDNA technology perceived the possibility of expressing *commercially* useful proteins in inexpensive bacteria cultures as part of their broader research agendas. Thus, for certain researchers, the lifting of the moratorium marked the beginning of a quest to produce higher organism proteins, such as insulin, in lower organisms, most notably the bacteria *E. coli*.[13]

RESEARCH COORDINATORS

This case study focuses upon research whose goal was the expression of human insulin in bacteria. Research of this sort was organized by a relatively small number of molecular biology and biochemistry labs. In Stephen Hall's popular account of the "race" to synthesize human insulin,[14] he divides the research activities into three groups. The groups' coordinators were Walter Gilbert, the team of William Rutter and Howard Goodman, and Herbert Boyer, respectively.[15] Organizing analysis of the insulin research by lab chief provides

---

[12]This is by no means an exhaustive review of the major advances that took place in the mid-1970s. Utilization of X-ray detection techniques, radioactive assays, and high-pressure liquid chromatography (HPLC) are just a few examples of the expanding array of tools and techniques available to the genetic researcher.

[13]It should be noted that the expression of commercially useful proteins in bacteria was *not* the direction pursued by most researchers. Further, university labs pursuing insulin expression in bacteria perceived the project as a "particular application" of the broader research program of the lab.

[14]The concept of a "race" is introduced here to reflect the tone and style of much of the published literature on the insulin research. The definition of a race, however, is ambiguous, and most analysis that examines investment races is imprecise as to what is driving the "overinvestment" in research (see, for example, Fudenberg et al., 1983).

[15] Other labs, for example, one at the University of Toronto, pursued rDNA insulin research, but Harvard, UCSF, and Genentech represent the most heavily invested and successful participants in this research.

sharp focus for identifying interdisciplinary and interinstitutional links. However, this focus comes at a cost. There is underemphasis on the influence and mobility of postdoctoral researchers and the degree of cooperation between the groups. However, providing the context and backgrounds of each of the principal labs will allow for the identification of crossover and cooperation later on.

Walter Gilbert's group worked primarily out of the Harvard Biology Labs. Gilbert, a physicist by training, was perhaps the most celebrated scientist to be involved in the insulin research. In the late 1960s, Gilbert completed seminal work on the *lac* repressor, providing important insights into the regulation of gene expression. Further, Gilbert was instrumental in the revolution in DNA sequencing in the mid-1970s. Gilbert maintained a large, active, and diverse lab at Harvard. Only a few of the research projects being pursued had direct bearing on the insulin research. Gilbert recalls that his lab was pursuing research on sequencing, genetic control mechanisms, and general methods for the expression of proteins in bacteria. He characterizes the insulin research as merely a specific application of these more general research themes (telephone interview on February 18, 1993, of Walter Gilbert, Professor, Department of Molecular Biology and Biochemistry, Harvard University, February 18, 1993).

The respective labs of Howard Goodman and William Rutter, both of UCSF, decided to collaborate on the insulin research. The collaboration was initiated because members of both labs were independently attempting to express rat insulin in *E. coli*. Rutter, chairman of biochemistry at UCSF during the 1970s, pursued the project as part of his lab's larger goal of exploring "differentiation of the pancreas" (telephone interview on June 14, 1993, of William Rutter, Professor of Biochemistry, University of California, San Francisco, and President, Chiron Corporation, June 14, 1993). Much of the research within Rutter's lab at the time "related in one way or another" to the insulin research. Indeed, expression of insulin was a particular and useful application of the projects being pursued by the lab at the time.[16] Howard Goodman, on the other hand, was a younger researcher with a smaller lab. Collaborative work with Herbert Boyer earlier in the decade had given Goodman's lab more experience with recombinant technology than Rutter's lab. Both labs were attempting to capitalize upon the new methods and technologies: "When it became evident that you could consider cloning . . . then it was obvious we should shift our program prominently, or even dominantly—and, as it turned out, almost solely—to the issues of isolating the genes as a prelude to finding out how they were expressed" (William Rutter, quoted in Hall, 1988, pp. 91–92).

---

[16] These projects included methods of cloning and expression, understanding of the enzymes involved in transcription, and the role of transfer ribonucleic acid in the regulation of intron/extron expression and recombination (telephone interview with Rutter, 1993).

Lastly, Herbert Boyer had organized a medium-size lab at UCSF. Boyer's lab was one of the most advanced recombinant technology labs in the world. In particular, Boyer's lab specialized in the construction of plasmids, also known as vectors. Vectors are the circular DNA material that can be easily transferred in and out of cells. Restriction enzymes developed by Boyer's lab resulted in a method for "cutting and pasting" DNA strands onto plasmid DNA. This method and the resulting vectors that could be easily manipulated, both fortes of Boyer's lab, were crucial components of the new gene-splicing technology.

Shortly before the NIH regulations were announced, though, Boyer's potential research base expanded. Along with Bob Swanson, a venture capitalist, Boyer formed Genentech,[17] the first biotechnology firm focused on recombinant DNA technologies.[18] Genentech, after an initial $1,000 investment split evenly between Boyer and Swanson, was initially capitalized by Kleiner & Perkins, a San Francisco-based venture capital firm for which Swanson had previously worked. The initial investment by Kleiner & Perkins was $100,000. Boyer's corporate affiliation affected the research activities of Boyer's lab—Genentech's first research contract was directly with Boyer's lab. Boyer and Swanson soon expanded the set of labs that Genentech invested in. Within nine months, Genentech contracted with researchers at City of Hope National Medical Center outside of Los Angeles to explore synthesis of a human gene.

These sketches are intended to provide a backdrop for understanding the research strategies and outcomes of each group. With the addition of a descriptive history of the research activities of each group, the interdisciplinary and interinstitutional links that were formed during this period can be examined and interpreted.

A SHORT HISTORY OF THE rDNA INSULIN RESEARCH PROJECTS

The expression of human insulin in bacteria was identified as a feasible research goal by the time that rDNA experimentation resumed in the summer of 1976. The most influential labs, equipped with a novel set of procedures, tools, and questions, attempted to carve out important but "doable" research projects. Projects were chosen that would allow for experimentation, refinement, and expansion of the developing technology as well as resolution of long-standing ques-

---

[17]The story of the founding of Genentech and the early interactions of Boyer and Swanson are well documented (e.g., Lewin, 1978).

[18] Cetus Corporation, located across the San Francisco Bay, had been in existence for nearly five years when Genentech was formed. Cetus' focus, however, was broader than that of Genentech, and Ronald Cape, Cetus' president, predicted that genetically engineered insulin was at least five years away as late as 1977.

tions in molecular biology and biochemistry. Insulin, a relatively small gene with interesting properties, was a prime candidate for a major lab's research agenda.

Expression of insulin in bacteria could be achieved by a number of distinct methods, namely, complementary DNA (cDNA) cloning, shotgunning, or synthesis.[19] The precise procedures, as well as the instrumentation, for each of these methods were still rudimentary. More importantly, each method revealed different types of *scientific* information. Complementary DNA cloning, by starting with messenger RNA (mRNA) as its source material, could provide far more insight than gene synthesis into questions of gene regulation, the interaction between DNA and mRNA, and the intergenerational transmission of genetic information. Artificial synthesis, by its very nature, merely mimicked human genetic information for the purpose of protein expression, rather than providing a vantage point for analysis of human genetic information. Researchers who were interested in exploring broader questions of biology, then, were biased in favor of cDNA methods. Not surprisingly, the Harvard and UCSF groups' insulin research revolved around cDNA methods, while Genentech, through contracts with City of Hope Medical Center, explored the possibilities of gene synthesis.

The first major milestone in the research was achieved by the Rutter-Goodman lab in early 1977. The goal of their research project was to insert the rat insulin gene into *E. coli*. The first task was to acquire a small amount of rat-derived, purified pancreatic RNA.[20] The rat pancreas RNA, laboriously distilled by a postdoctoral researcher in Rutter's lab, John Chirgwin, provided the UCSF researchers with the important intermediate genetic material that provides a transcription of the rat's genetic code. Alex Ullrich, a postdoctoral researcher in Goodman's lab, then "backwards-engineered" the MRNA into the original DNA strands utilizing *reverse transcriptase*.[21] These DNA strands were then spliced into a plasmid utilizing the Cohen-Boyer technique. The vector was then in-

---

[19]It may be instructive to note that cDNA cloning, the most elegant method for isolation, begins with messenger RNA (mRNA) as source material and, utilizing reverse transcriptase, "backs out" the original DNA sequence. Shotgunning, a more cumbersome method useful for obtaining simple genetic structures from lower organisms, requires cutting up an organism's entire genome, inserting plasmids into bacteria, and isolating those bacteria that ended up receiving plasmids that contain the sought-after DNA. Synthesis, as described above, entails the construction of a gene by stringing together nucleotides in the appropriate order. Sylvester and Klotz (1983) provide a readable introduction to the techniques of genetic engineering.

[20]More precisely, the cDNA technique utilized required the isolation of mRNA, the intermediate genetic material that transports instructions from DNA to a ribosome for the purpose of protein production.

[21]Reverse transcriptase is a type of enzyme discovered by David Baltimore that catalyzes the production of DNA strands in interaction mRNA.

serted into *E. coli*. Finally, the plasmid DNA of the *E. coli* was sequenced, indicating that a portion of the *E. coli* colony did, indeed, possess the genetic material for rat insulin (Ullrich et al., 1977).

To put the experiment in perspective, the insertion of a eukaryotic gene into *E. coli* had been achieved as early as 1974 (Morrow et al., 1974), and the procedure for doing so would be commonplace by the early 1980s. On the other hand, Ullrich and Chirgwin achieved substantial innovation in terms of the sophistication and reliability of the cDNA cloning procedure. According to Hall (1988, p. 140), "The suite of techniques they put together while cloning insulin instantly became a how-to manual for molecular biologists all over the world." Further, the experiment represented the first time a medically useful gene was successfully inserted into bacteria. The experiment highlighted the potential of the new techniques while simultaneously focusing upon insulin as a studiable hormone.

Nearly six months after the experiment's publication in *Science* (Ullrich et al., 1977), it was disclosed that the UCSF researchers had broken NIH guidelines during their research (Wade, 1977). In particular, while the *Science* paper reported research that utilized the vector pMB9 in April 1977, the research team had previously attempted the experiment in January of the same year with another vector, pBR322.[22] Both vectors, products of Herbert Boyer's lab, were required to be reviewed, approved, and certified by the Recombinant DNA Advisory Committee (RAC) prior to their use in experiments. While pBR322 had been approved by RAC, it had not yet been *certified*, the necessary condition for using the plasmid for the experiment. Whether or not Ullrich, the principal cloner in the experiment, recognized his use of pBR322 as a violation of NIH policy is unclear; contemporary discussion allowed for the possibility of an honest mistake (Wade, 1977). When the violation was brought to the attention of lab director William Rutter, the work was halted, though not officially disclosed to NIH.[23] Two months later, when pMB9, another acceptable plasmid for the experiment, was certified, the experiment was repeated and was successful. On the basis of this later work, the group published their findings in *Science*, holding a press conference three weeks before publication. The *Science* article that disclosed the violation gives a negative view of the UCSF researchers: "Capitalism sticking its nose in the lab has tainted interpersonal relations—there are a number of people who feel rather strongly that there should be no commercialization of human insulin" (David Martin, quoted in Wade, 1977, p. 1342). Further, the

---

[22]Vectors, such as pMB9 or pBR322, were named by their "creators," in this case, Mary Betlach (MB) and Bolivar and Rodriguez (BR), respectively.

[23]There was informal contact with NIH concerning the violation of RAC rules. However, there was no formal procedure with NIH, nor did the group volunteer the information in the original *Science* paper or in the press conference that announced the results of the research (Hall, 1988, pp. 134–144).

article noted that "The UCSF team was in competition with a group at Harvard which was known to be working with a better source material" (Wade, 1977, p. 1342). The exposé highlights both competition between labs for scientific primacy and the potential commercial applications of the insulin research. The UCSF experiment was of interest to both the academic and commercial community. True, the UCSF researchers were still far from expressing human insulin in bacteria; but the experimental steps towards that goal were now far more clear. Conversely, understanding of gene regulation and expression was still developing, and the insertion experiment provided important tools for this basic research agenda.

While both the Goodman-Rutter collaborators and the Gilbert group experimented with insertion and expression of the rat insulin gene, Genentech contracted with researchers for the purpose of refining and expanding upon methods of gene synthesis and expression. Genentech contracted with Herbert Boyer's own gene cloning and plasmid construction lab at UCSF, as well as with Arthur Riggs and Keiichi Itakura of City of Hope National Medical Center just outside of Los Angeles. Upon the advice and requests of Riggs and Itakura, Genentech funded experiments whose goal was the expression of synthetic somatostatin, a simpler human hormone than insulin.[24] While somatostatin was not perceived to have any direct commercial value, it was viewed by its Genentech funders as an acceptable first step toward the synthesis of the insulin gene. Itakura's goal in synthesizing somatostatin was to improve upon, refine, and expand the Khorana technique announced in early 1976. Itakura's technique reduced the time necessary for the synthesis procedure from years to weeks. While building upon the group's earlier research,[25] the somatostatin project provided an opportunity to standardize procedures as well as build up a library of "codons," nucleotide triples that are translated into the intracellular production of an amino acid.[26]

By early 1977, Itakura, refining his method, was able to produce purified somatostatin DNA. To clone and express the gene, artificial somatostatin genes

---

[24]Riggs and Itakura, while negotiating with Boyer and Swanson, also applied to NIH for funding of the same project. The grant request was turned down on the basis of its lack of applicability (Hall, 1988, p. 83).

[25]The group's earlier "non-Genentech-funded" collaboration involved the synthesis and insertion of the *lac* operator, a small strand of genetic material that regulates expression. The research team, headed by Itakura and Riggs at City of Hope, included Boyer, Herbert Heynekker, John Goodman, and John Shine of UCSF, as well as researchers from the California Institute of Technology and the University of Ottawa. Ironically, the experiment was inspired by Walter Gilbert, who suggested a critical experimental technique. Thus, the *lac* operator experiment involved collaboration by researchers in all three of the distinct research teams involved in the insulin research.

[26]Similar to Khorana's research, Itakura's utilized commercially available chemicals to construct DNA strands. The speed of the synthetic method greatly increased as the number of ready-made codons increased. To provide context, the expression of a protein (such as the insulin hormone) involves the production of a specific sequence of amino acids that "fold" to create the desired protein.

were sent to Boyer's UCSF lab. Herb Heyneker, a postdocoral researcher in the lab, spliced the gene into pBR322, the same vector as used in the rat insulin experiment. The vector was then inserted into *E. coli*. By August 1977, the team had expressed somatostatin in bacteria. The experiment marked the first instance of expression of a human protein in bacteria. For this alone, the somatostatin experiment represented a milestone in rDNA research. However, Itakura's technique and tools proved to be widely applicable to other problems within biochemistry.[27]

Once made practical by Itakura, genetic synthesis possessed an important advantage over cDNA cloning: cloning with synthetic material was not covered by RAC guidelines.[28] Thus, in contrast to cDNA research, which often required expensive and time-consuming precautions, the Genentech researchers only had to obey minimal safety precautions. For research on nonhuman genetic material, this difference was mostly one of convenience. The rat insulin experiments, for example, were conducted in a lab that required close containment of air, changing one's clothes, and a closely monitored waste disposal process. Research on natural human genetic material, however, required extraordinary precautions. Military biowarfare labs were the only facilities with adequate biological and physical containment to pass RAC guidelines for experiments with human genetic material (P4 facilities). Access to these facilities was extremely rare and difficult to obtain. Complementary DNA cloning of human genetic material could be halted, in essence, because of the strict RAC guidelines. Genentech researchers, pursuing the synthetic approach, faced no such regulatory constraints.

Much of the scientific insight from cDNA cloning did not require the use of natural human genetic material, however. The Gilbert group at Harvard continued to pursue expression of rat insulin in bacteria. The Gilbert group's goal was to modify the insertion procedure of Ullrich (of the Rutter-Goodman group) to achieve expression of rat insulin. Argiris Efstratiadis, a postdoctoral researcher in the lab of Fotis Kafatos, attempted to produce the cDNA gene. Efstratiadis worked with RNA from pancreatic rat tumors developed by William Chick of the Harvard Medical School. Efstratiadis' goal was to purify the RNA extracted from the tumors, and "backwards-engineer" the rat insulin DNA strands. Forrest Fuller, of Gilbert's lab, attempted to develop a method of inserting the cDNA strand into bacteria in such a way that the bacteria would start manufacturing insulin.

The insulin research supervised by Gilbert was less successful than the Rutter-Goodman researchers for meeting the goal of successful insertion of the

---

[27]Itakura's results are widely cited in the explanation of the emerging techniques (Cohen, 1982, p. 25).

[28]See footnote 7.

gene. Further, Fuller, a graduate student, worked unsuccessfully with globin[29] as Efstratiadis could not yet provide the rat insulin gene. Perhaps more telling, Fuller was forced, at the request of Gilbert, to leave the Gilbert lab at the end of 1977, just six months after the UCSF insulin research was published in *Science*.[30] Fuller's approach to gene expression was discarded, and Gilbert recruited Lydia Villa-Komaroff, a more experienced postdoctoral researcher in Fotis Kafatos' lab, to be responsible for cloning and expression in the insulin research. In addition, Stephanie Broome, another graduate student in Gilbert's lab, provided a detection technique that allowed the Harvard researchers to recognize even minute amounts of protein expression.

Within six months of formulating the new research plan,[31] the Harvard group achieved expression of rat insulin in bacteria. Moreover, the bacteria *secreted* the rat insulin. The secretion of protein from bacteria was an unintended by-product of the experimental strategy, but it was not without value. More specifically, the expression of mammalian protein in bacteria by cDNA cloning represented an important scientific contribution, while the resulting secretion of protein provided clear-cut possibilities for commercial application. The paper reporting the results (Villa-Komaroff et al., 1978) is widely cited as a seminal work in gene expression, while Harvard's patent is a broad claim over techniques that involve protein secretion in bacteria.

Consequently, by the summer of 1978, two alternative methods for expressing human insulin in bacteria seemed feasible: cDNA cloning and chemical synthesis. Moreover, each research group designed a strategy that, if successful, would result in expression. Expression of human insulin in bacteria represented the first important commercial application of rDNA technology. Not surprisingly, then, the level of interest by the pharmaceutical and investment communities increased as these strategies were formulated. The Rutter-Goodman researchers, the Gilbert group, and the Genentech researchers funded human insulin experiments with private (corporate) funds. Genentech, by construction, utilized venture capital to fund research. Not surprisingly, the success of the somatostatin experiment had considerably increased the level of financing available to Genentech. For expression of human insulin, Genentech was able to establish its own laboratory in South San Francisco and hire its first full-time researchers, Dennis Kleid and David Goeddel. The Harvard researchers, in contrast, reached

---

[29]Globin is an essential protein in the construction of red blood cells and had been utilized by the Harvard researchers in earlier research.

[30]Stephen Hall's account of the dismissal of Forrest Fuller highlights the trade-off that Gilbert faced between the successful execution of the insulin research and the successful training of Fuller as a graduate student (Hall, 1988, pp. 176–178).

[31]Their research plan included a novel proposal for the placement of the gene along the plasmid pBR322, which allowed for easier identification of the bacteria colonies where the rat insulin would be expressed.

a funding agreement with Biogen, a new, internationally oriented biotechnology start-up firm. Gilbert, as a celebrated scientist, had been courted by Biogen's founders and had agreed to chair its scientific advisory board.[32] Within weeks of the announcement of the rat insulin expression experiment, a funding agreement had been reached between Gilbert's lab and Biogen for research on expression of human insulin. Finally, in August 1978, the Rutter-Goodman labs finalized a complex funding arrangement with Eli Lilly. The Lilly research contract included research on insulin and human growth hormone, among other products. The UCSF researchers involved in the rat insulin insertion experiment, most notably Alex Ullrich, agreed with Lilly to pursue research on expression of human insulin.[33]

By focusing on the expression of human genetic material, those researchers utilizing cDNA cloning methods were required to satisfy far more stringent RAC guidelines than were necessary for the rat insulin experiments. As mentioned earlier, very few locations possessed sufficient safety precautions to satisfy the regulation, and most of the acceptable locations were military biowarfare labs. Indeed, both the Gilbert group and Alex Ullrich were forced to leave the United States in order to conduct experiments on human insulin. As discussed below, Lilly arranged for Ullrich to work in France, where regulation concerning containment was slightly more lax; Gilbert, utilizing Biogen connections, secured a month-long research stay at England's Porton Down Microbiology Research Labs, a military research center. Genentech researchers, in contrast, were able to operate their cloning operations out of a leased warehouse in South San Francisco.

The UCSF insulin effort was the one least focused on direct commercial application. During the summer of 1978, Ullrich continued to work with rat genetic material to achieve two aims: expression of rat insulin in bacteria through cDNA cloning and the isolation and sequencing of the chromosomal rat gene. The first goal reflected an interest in mastering and refining the techniques for expression and secretion demonstrated by the Harvard group earlier that year. The isolation of chromosomal insulin DNA, on the other hand, would result in the ability to read the entirety of the insulin gene, *even those strands that are not transcribed into RNA.*[34] Ullrich's insulin research was aligned with Lilly's fund-

---

[32]Gilbert would later leave his post at Harvard to become president of Biogen. Because of difficulties in bringing products to market, Gilbert was replaced by the board of Biogen, and he returned to Harvard in 1984 (Hall, 1988, pp. 315–316).

[33]John Seeburg, another postdoctoral researcher in Goodman's lab, was the primary researcher on human growth hormone.

[34]The important distinction here is between the identification of exons, genetic material that is expressed, and introns, genetic material that is spliced out during translation into RNA. While this distinction is not critical for the analysis here, the importance of the intron/exon distinction was a "hot" topic in molecular biology at the time and Ullrich's shotgunning approach to finding insulin provided a method for reading both the intron and exon regions of the insulin gene.

ing goals. Thus, shortly after the UCSF-Lilly funding agreement was finalized, Ullrich traveled to a Lilly facility in France where experiments with human genetic material could be conducted. Ullrich's research efforts in France were unsuccessful, in part because of accidental contamination of his experimental materials during travel. However, even if Ullrich had been successful in reaching his short-term research goals during the France trip, he would not have achieved expression of human insulin before the Genentech researchers.

During his time in France, Ullrich decided to disassociate himself from the Goodman lab. After the insertion experiment, the hostility and antagonism between Ullrich and his lab director, Howard Goodman, had steadily increased. The sources of the antagonism were numerous: disagreements over scientific credit, conflicts over patent recognition, the provision of adequate lab support, the insertion experiment's "plasmid" episode, and personal antipathy.[35] Along with his lab colleague, Peter Seeburg, Ullrich accepted a long-standing offer of employment from Bob Swanson of Genentech. Genentech thus hired two of the most talented postdoctoral researchers of the Rutter-Goodman labs.

Gilbert's group, in contrast to the UCSF researchers, was intent on the expression of human insulin during the summer and early autumn of 1978. Four Harvard researchers, Gilbert, Efstratiadis, Villa-Komaroff, and Broome,[36] secured a one-month research stay at Porton Down Microbiology Research Labs in England. The trip and research were funded by Biogen. The goal of the trip was to express human insulin in bacteria utilizing the same experimental strategy that had been successful with the rat gene. Like Ullrich, unfortunately, there was a serious contamination of the group's source material during their preparations for travel. The contamination was only discovered after substantial experimentation at Porton Down. Moreover, their research stay was not long enough to salvage the experiment. If the research at Porton Down had been successful, the Gilbert group may have had a chance of expressing insulin in bacteria roughly contemporaneously with the Genentech team. Instead, the Gilbert group, and Biogen, were unsuccessful in their goal of commercializing the insulin research of the late 1970s.

This is not to say that additional scientific research was not pursued by the Harvard lab on the insulin gene; insulin, as a "studiable" gene, remained an important focus of inquiry for molecular biologists. Nor did Gilbert, or Biogen, cease to attempt commercial exploitation of the insulin gene. In fact, in 1981, Biogen contracted with Novo Industri, the second largest insulin manufacturer in

---

[35]Hall provides detailed evidence of personal antagonisms within the UCSF lab (Hall, 1988, pp. 204–207, 277–283).

[36]Efstratiadis and Villa-Komaroff, having been hired as assistant professors, were in the process of moving to Harvard Medical School and the University of Massachusetts Medical Center, respectively.

the world, to develop a process for cloning human insulin. While this research was not entirely successful, it did provide Biogen with income before its public offering. However, the lack of success at Porton Down, and Genentech's contemporaneous success in California, substantially reduced the financial benefits to Harvard and to Gilbert of the insulin research.

Genentech, on the other hand, achieved a large measure of corporate security with the expression of human insulin in the summer of 1978. A research contract, ensuring a steady stream of income, was negotiated with Eli Lilly after the successful achievement of expression of human insulin in bacteria. The research strategy utilized mirrored the somatostatin project, though additional players were brought onto the team, such as David Goeddel and Dennis Kleid, for the actual cloning. The experience with somatostatin also provided important solutions to problems facing the team: "When we started the insulin project, DNA synthesis was not the risky part. We were improving on . . . work on the somatostatin project" (telephone interview on February 18, 1993, of Keiichi Itakura, Department of Molecular Genetics, City of Hope National Medical Center, February 18, 1993).

Insulin, however, was a more complicated gene than somatostatin. Achieving expression required the development of a series of innovative techniques. The first difficulty involved the construction of the separate chains of DNA that together form insulin. Pancreatic production of insulin involves three chains, the A, B, and C chains, where only amino acids from the A and B chains are actually present in insulin. The C chain links the A and B chain and is "snipped" off as it links the two chains. Goeddel, working with Itakura's team at City of Hope, first had to assemble the A and B chains separately and insert them into appropriate plasmids. The B chain, however, was cleaved into two sections, to allow for easier manipulation and reduce risk of failure during synthesis or expression. The second difficulty was *reconstitution*, the process by which the A chain and B chain were to be linked together. The reconstitution procedure, regarded as somewhat doubtful in and of itself, required extensive purification of the insulin chains. The purification was achieved by the repeated use of HPLC (high-performance liquid chromatography), an efficient distilling method which had gained increased popularity during the 1970s. Reconstituted, the A and B chains formed insulin. The last hurdle overcome by the Genentech researchers was the requirement that the insulin produced be efficiently "harvested" for commercial use. This was not easy, as the method of inserting the insulin gene into bacteria required that the insulin expressed be bonded with another protein, betagalactosidase (beta-gal). Arthur Riggs constructed a breakable methionine link between the beta-gal molecule and the insulin molecule which allowed for the separation of insulin and beta-gal. This innovation allowed the harvesting of pure insulin. While this technique was obviously refined during scale-up, Riggs' procedure significantly advanced the commercialization prospects of the Genentech effort. In contrast, the Gilbert group, even if they had been successful in the expression experiment, would have been much farther away from commercialization than the Genentech effort. Once these experimental barriers were overcome, a radioactive assay was utilized to detect the presence of human insulin within bacteria. On August 24, 1978, the Genentech team, working at City of Hope, successfully expressed human insulin in bacteria.

Obviously, the Genentech result did not mark the end of research on insulin, either in a scientific or in a commercial sense. Both the Rutter-Goodman labs, as well the Gilbert lab, continued to explore the scientific properties of insulin. One of the principal results of that research was the isolation and sequencing of the chromosomal human insulin gene in late 1979. Isolation of the rat insulin gene provided key insights into the interaction between introns, exons, and the modes of intergenerational transmissions of genetic information.

On the commercial side, Genentech and Eli Lilly signed a research and royalty agreement shortly after the Genentech expression experiment. Each contributed toward the scale-up program associated with the production of rDNA insulin. Genentech researchers spent much of 1979 increasing the insulin yields from *E. coli*. One of the most important Genentech innovations of this period was the introduction of the *trp* system. When insulin was first expressed, the experimental procedure required each of the insulin chains to be linked to beta-gal. Unfortunately, beta-gal was an extremely large molecule, and for each molecule of insulin produced, a molecule of beta-gal had to be produced. The large size of beta-gal decreased the potential yield of insulin from each bacterial cell. The *trp* system, in contrast, utilized a much smaller bacterial enzyme, *trp* E, which had the additional advantage of being easier to manipulate.

Once the Genentech yields were sufficiently high, Lilly began the construction of pilot plants in expectation of commercial production. Lilly also managed the complicated process of FDA approval. Extensive pharmacological experience with beef and pork insulin, however, decreased the regulatory burden. Humulin, Lilly's trade name for synthetic insulin, was first sold in 1983. To put perspective on the importance of the introduced method, Humulin sales now account for over 60 percent of the sales in the domestic U.S. insulin market ($300 million).

In sum, this case study provides an intimate view of the university-industry interface with respect to medical innovation. Humulin, while the most visible, is only one of the end products of the research recounted here. An array of techniques, refined tools, and scientific insights emerged as a result of this research and have been steadily built upon for both scientific and commercial exploitation.

THE ROLE OF INTERDISCIPLINARY RESEARCH

The insulin research was not only interdisciplinary; the experiments reshaped the boundaries of existing disciplines. While genetic engineering is most often linked with molecular biology, the insulin research involved organic chemists, a diverse group of pancreatic researchers, and biochemists. Moreover, the insulin research, in conjunction with contemporaneous rDNA research, transformed the practice of biochemistry in general, aligning it more closely with the methodology and techniques of molecular biology.

Biochemistry and Molecular Biology

The links between biochemistry and molecular biology are the most salient place to begin analysis of interdisciplinary forces in this case study. The critical differences between biochemistry and molecular biology are actually a matter of debate and have certainly changed over time. As mentioned above, Paul Berg claims that molecular biology was an approach and philosophy toward bioresearch adopted by an increasing number of experimenters during the 1970s, and that the increase in this adoption was partially a function of the increasing availability of tools and technology (telephone interview with Paul Berg, Professor of Biochemistry, Stanford University, February 17, 1993). Gilbert, on the other hand, notes that while particular distinctions do not do justice to the set of skills possessed by a researcher in either field, biochemists might be more interested in activities such as the purification of proteins while molecular biologists would be more interested in the manipulation of DNA through the use of enzymes (telephone interview with Walter Gilbert, Professor, Department of Molecular Biology and Biochemistry, Harvard University, February 18, 1993).

Irrespective of definition, the insulin research sat clearly between the two disciplines. Moreover, the insulin research[37] provided a framework for interaction between researchers. The alliance between the labs of Rutter and Goodman, discussed earlier, amply demonstrates the point. Rutter's lab was more specialized in biochemistry, while Goodman's lab contained a set of talented molecular biologists. Members of each lab provided critical inputs into the research process. For example, Ullrich's success in the insertion experiment was crucially dependent on the isolation and purification of mRNA insulin from rats. The purification process, which could not have been adequately achieved by any member of the Goodman lab, was beautifully handled by John Chirgwin, a member of Rutter's lab. These interactions led to the transmission of information between researchers from the two labs. Thus, for future research, the biochemists in Rutter's lab were able to leverage the new techniques of genetic engineering, while molecular biologists such as Ullrich became more acquainted with the techniques of purification. The application of molecular biology to insulin research resulted in an expansion of the skill base of both biochemists and molecular biologists.

---

[37]Along with other work (e.g., human growth hormone).

Organic Chemistry and Molecular Biology

Organic chemistry played an important, though not clearly foreseeable, role in the insulin research. Keiichi Itakura, the principal organic chemist working for Genentech, claims (somewhat exaggeratedly) that "99.9 percent of organic chemists work on other and different topics; 0.1 percent of organic chemists work on DNA synthesis" (telephone interview with Keiichi Itakura, Department of Molecular Genetics, City of Hope National Medical Center, February 18, 1993). In other words, the proper role for an organic chemist in genetic engineering research was not obvious before the insulin research. Itakura perceived the opportunity to make synthesis a common tool in genetic engineering. As a consequence, the impact of Itakura's research was felt most pointedly in molecular biology and biochemistry, rather than organic chemistry. This research focus for Itakura involved professional risk. If the synthetic approach had not been susceptible to improvement, Itakura's reputation as an organic chemist would have been marginal (as DNA chemistry was only a small part of organic chemistry) while his work would have failed as a useful *application* of organic chemistry to another discipline. As it was, Itakura's success ensured his standing within the organic chemistry community as well as the more general scientific community.

In contrast to biochemists who pursued the insulin research in order to acquire experience with the emerging tools of molecular biology, Itakura specialized in chemical synthesis and did not deal directly with gene splicing or expression. Itakura recalls that molecular biologists were responsible for "handling DNA molecules" (telephone interview, K. Itakura, 1993). This contrast highlights the direction of interaction. Where Itakura's chemistry served as an input into genetic engineering, molecular biologists and biochemists informed each other by expanding each others' knowledge and providing novel contexts for applications.

Interactions with the Wider Medical and Scientific Community

Researchers into rDNA insulin also interacted with the more general medical community (and pancreatic researchers in particular). Expression of insulin in bacteria required the knowledge and resources of individuals who were knowledgeable about insulin. Both the Harvard and UCSF researchers acquired this information through the formation of a research relationship with a researcher in their respective medical schools.

The Gilbert group teamed up with William Chick, a researcher at the Harvard Medical School. Chick's research on the inducement of rat insulin tumors yielded rich source material for the Harvard researchers. Chick's contribution was quite critical—Harvard's "better source material" is mentioned in the *Science* article that exposed the use of an uncertified vector in the UCSF insertion experiment (Wade, 1977).

Rutter and Goodman allied themselves with John Baxter, who was a member of both the biochemistry department and the medical clinic at UCSF. While Baxter's role within the insulin research reviewed in this case study was small, he collaborated with the Rutter-Goodman labs on human growth hormone. Growth hormone, like insulin, was being aggressively pursued by molecular biologists at this time (McKelvey, 1993). Moreover, Baxter's lab was included in the research agreement that was reached with Eli Lilly in August 1978. Baxter provided the most direct link from the Rutter-Goodman labs to the more general medical community.

Finally, the role of *multidisciplinary*, as opposed to *interdisciplinary*, researchers should be highlighted. While most components of the research involved collaboration between researchers from different fields, there is a notable example within the insulin research of a researcher crossing fields. Walter Gilbert's graduate school training was in physics, as was his first faculty appointment. His entree into molecular biology was the result of persistent encouragement by James Watson during the late 1950s. While the migration of physicists into other scientific fields has been examined elsewhere (Rosenberg, 1992), it is almost ironic that Gilbert, the ex-physicist, would enter a field, molecular biology, that itself would dramatically redefine the boundaries and priorities of a wide range of disciplines.

The Nature of Interdisciplinary Research

Defining disciplinary goals and demonstrating the interactions between researchers from different disciplines provides a pedagogically sound mapping of the terrain. However, the deeper insight is best stated by Walter Gilbert: "When one is working on the frontier, nearly anything that one puts one's fingerprint on will be interdisciplinary" (telephone interview with Walter Gilbert, Professor, Department of Molecular Biology and Biochemistry, Harvard University, February 18, 1993). Only a small number of researchers had mastered the emerging techniques of genetic engineering at the time of this case study. The general excitement within this small community and the feeling by researchers that they were breaking important new scientific ground with commercial application diminished the importance of disciplinary boundaries. Moreover, successful research resulted from the mastering of techniques and tools. Indeed, advances in molecular biology led to potential consequences in scientific sectors distant from molecular biology. The difficulty of acquiring the skills to mine this potential, along with the prestige to be had by mining it, resulted in a curious but consequential collection of collaborations and crossovers.

THE ROLE OF INTERINSTITUTIONAL RESEARCH

Interinstitutional collaboration and linkage is ubiquitous in the insulin research programs. In particular, each group utilized private funding during their research as well as forming collaborations between researchers at different academic institutions. Additionally, Genentech's willingness to form these types of partnerships was markedly more pronounced than that of the Harvard or UCSF groups.

Academic Collaboration

The Gilbert and Rutter-Goodman groups seem to have shared a common model for collaboration and interinstitutional interaction. With respect to academic collaborations, each group attempted to limit the number of links formed during the research project. This is not to say that links were not formed. Instead, links were formed only after it became apparent that a particular set of characteristics were present in a proposed collaboration. William Rutter notes three of these characteristics: "complementing your own research objective," "believing you will get an answer faster," and introducing "specific expertise" (telephone interview with William Rutter, Professor of Biochemistry, University of California, San Francisco, and President, Chiron Corporation, June 14, 1993). For example, the UCSF group pursued, for a while, a collaboration with researchers at the University of Texas (most notably Peter Lomedico). The University of Texas researchers were supposed to assist with the acquisition of purified bovine insulin mRNA (telephone interview, W. Rutter, 1993). The UCSF research was stalled owing to the lack of source material for experiments and the link with the University of Texas was aimed at overcoming this fundamental obstacle in pursuing the research.

The Gilbert team's makeup also highlights the trade-offs associated with collaboration, albeit in a more subtle fashion. As discussed earlier, Gilbert first pursued the insulin research with Forrest Fuller, a graduate student in Gilbert's lab. While Fuller refined his cloning approach, the progress of the group's insulin research lagged. Gilbert, while supportive of Fuller's lack of experience during early stages of the research, eventually withdrew support for him. Argiris Efstratiadis then recruited Lydia Villa-Komaroff, a more seasoned postdoctoral cloner, to complete the project. This change in personnel clearly benefited the pace of the research, as the group achieved expression and secretion of rat insulin within six months. More significantly, however, the incident highlights the trade-off between the training of graduate students and the successful execution of important research. Gilbert preferred to align his own research goals with the training of his graduate students but, when this arrangement turned out to be unsuccessful, Gilbert collaborated with a more experienced specialist.

Genentech's willingness to cross institutional boundaries provides a striking contrast to the tactics of the other researchers. Indeed, the corporation was formed for exactly that purpose. Thus, the Genentech strategy relied on research at City of Hope, Boyer's UCSF lab, and its in-house lab consisting of Dennis Kleid and David Goeddel. While this increased willingness to cross institutional boundaries is not surprising, it is a distinctive feature of the successful Genentech strategy (and other small start-up firms). For example, the final tasks of the insulin research were divided between the City of Hope researchers and the Genentech researchers, Kleid and Goeddel. For a period of time, material was being shipped back and forth between northern and southern California. While this constituted a logical division of labor, Genentech's corporate funders believed the work could be speeded up by merging the two teams in one location. The two Genentech scientists were told, "You're going down to the City of Hope. Don't come back until it's done" (Bob Swanson, paraphrased by David Goeddel and quoted in Hall, 1988, p. 246). Indeed, the corporate form provides clear incentives to coordinate research among institutions with the goal of producing an appropriable product or process.

Financial Linkages

In addition to interinstitutional research collaborations, each of the research groups arranged for private funding of the insulin research. Both the Harvard and UCSF researchers arranged research funding agreements during the summer of 1978 (with Biogen and Eli Lilly, respectively). In contrast, the Genentech effort, by definition, was founded upon the infusion of private funding.

Once again, there are strong similarities between the Harvard and UCSF teams. Both pursued private funding relationships when their experimental strategy began to focus on human genetic material and the possibility of patentable and appropriable products and processes. In contrast, Genentech funders, whose sole goal was the development of appropriable products and processes, funded the somatostatin experiments, which had negligible economic value.

Further, one of the motivations for pursuing private funding by the university-based researchers was the possibility of acquiring access to facilities in which experiments with human genetic material was approved (P4 laboratories; see footnote 7). Indeed, as discussed above, the Gilbert group arranged their stay at Porton Down through Biogen connections, and Alex Ullrich completed a stay at Eli Lilly's French research facility. These connections were critical for these researchers, as there were very few sites at which experiments with human genetic material could be conducted. For the Harvard and UCSF researchers (and their funders), the RAC guidelines were burdensome and costly. By comparison, the Genentech strategy, which evaded RAC guidelines through the use of synthetic material, not only allowed the researchers greater freedom but reduced the cost of the research to the funders.

In sum, the types of interinstitutional links that were formed reveal sharp distinctions between the approaches of the Genentech researchers and the academic researchers. First, the willingness to form research collaborations was more prevalent among Genentech researchers. Secondly, the goals of Genentech researchers and their funders were more tightly aligned. In addition, strategies that aided in maintaining this close alignment of goals were spelled out early on (during the somatostatin experiments). As a consequence, the Genentech research strategy required few adjustments as the expression of human insulin became more feasible. In contrast, the Harvard and UCSF researchers needed to alter their funding arrangements as well as their base of operation as soon as they began experiments with human genetic material.

ANALYSIS AND CONCLUSIONS

This case study has focused upon rDNA insulin research in the late 1970s. In particular, the first three sections outlined the context and history of the insulin research. The next two sections examined the interdisciplinary and interinstitutional links which were formed during the experiments. These links were focused upon because they reveal sharp distinctions between the research strategies of the different research groups. In this concluding section, this heterogeneity is analyzed more systematically. The incentives to form these links are characterized, the cluster of characteristics that mark the research groups are identified, and the phenomena of interlab competition are addressed. Finally, the role of the insulin research in shaping future university-industry relationships is explored. This concluding section highlights our underlying query: Why do biotechnology firms and universities regard each other as complements, and is this relationship the result of the particular historical sequence that marked the early days of biotechnology?

The Existence of Heterogeneous Incentives

The three teams examined chose substantively different strategies for pursuing their research goals. More precisely, there are more similarities between the Gilbert and Rutter-Goodman groups than between these groups and the Genentech researchers. This dichotomy is apparent in the research strategies that were pursued, as well as in the interdisciplinary and interinstitutional links that were formed. One can understand these differences as the consequences of variation in the incentives faced by the different researchers. Simply put, Genentech faced very different incentives than either the Gilbert or Rutter-Goodman teams. Moreover, the two academically based teams faced quite similar incentive structures.

The primary difference between the incentives of the Genentech group and the academic groups is the degree to which trade-offs existed between the development of an appropriate product or process and other goals of the lab and its researchers. Genentech's very existence depended upon the successful completion of the insulin research project. While the development of novel scientific knowledge was a benefit of the research, the researchers were consistently focused on the expression of insulin in bacteria for the purpose of acquiring a royalty contract with a large pharmaceutical manufacturer. As the researchers closed in on this goal, ever greater organizational resources (both personal and financial) were invested with the sole purpose of bringing the project to fruition. Genentech, by its very design, was relatively unfettered by concerns other than the expression of insulin.

The Gilbert and Rutter-Goodman groups, in contrast, performed the research in an academic environment. Consequently, the research organizers needed to balance a multitude of goals. As academic researchers, they had incentives to utilize the insulin research for financial gain, but they also had responsibilities and incentives to train graduate and postdoctoral students as well as place the insulin research within the context of their broader scientific agenda. For example, while the Harvard effort was pushed by Walter Gilbert in particular directions, Gilbert notes that "we were limited by the practicalities of what graduate students and postdocs were interested in" (telephone interview with Walter Gilbert, Professor, Department of Molecular Biology and Biochemistry, Harvard University, February 18, 1993). Additionally, the insulin research at the academic labs was conducted with a set of *biological* questions in mind.[38] These restrictions did not bind Genentech. Instead, Swanson and Boyer were free to search for a lab where the insulin project could be carried out efficiently and without concern about tailoring the experimental strategy to reveal information of scientific importance.

The contrast between the incentives faced by Genentech and the academic researchers increased as the research neared completion. As mentioned above, Genentech had incentives to become consistently more focused on the sole goal of insulin expression as the research proceeded. The Harvard and UCSF groups had difficulties achieving a comfortable balance. At Harvard, Gilbert decided to discontinue support for his graduate student, Forrest Fuller, in order to maintain the pace of his insulin research. The UCSF group experienced even greater difficulties in balancing the competing objectives of different researchers. Howard Goodman, in particular, was widely credited with assembling a talented group of molecular biologists, but with failing to adequately support and reward his researchers during their research (Hall, 1988, p. 206). In fact, as mentioned earlier, shortly after Genentech successfully cloned insulin two of Goodman's best postdoctoral researchers accepted employment offers from Genentech.[39] These difficulties at UCSF are attributable, at least in part, to the need by the lab to balance a complex set of competing objectives.

---

[38]Rutter, Gilbert, and Efstratiadis all mention scientific goals as their motivations. For example, how is gene expression regulated? What were the roles of introns and exons? For William Rutter, a pancreatic researcher, one of the principal research queries was "what are the intracellular processes of pancreatic beta cells which allow the body to produce insulin?" Note that these questions are only peripherally related to the expression of *human* insulin in bacteria, particularly when the experiments are being guided by an eventual goal of commercial production.

[39]Alex Ullrich and Peter Seeburg.

The Consequences of Heterogeneous Incentives

Because the research groups faced different incentives, their experimental strategies, as well as their willingness to form interdisciplinary and interinstitutional links, were quite different. In fact, by contrasting researchers with dissimilar incentives, clusters of strategic characteristics can be identified which highlight the manner in which researchers responded to the idiosyncratic set of incentives that they face.

The most salient features of the Genentech strategy were the pressure to achieve expression of insulin quickly (and publicly), the desire to avoid costly regulatory barriers, and the willingness to form an eclectic set of interdisciplinary and interinstitutional links. The decision to pursue chemical synthesis of the gene (rather than cDNA cloning) is an important manifestation of this strategy. Though important scientifically, chemical synthesis "was a chemical challenge, not a biological challenge" (telephone interview with William Rutter, Professor of Biochemistry, University of California, San Francisco, and President, Chiron Corporation, June 14, 1993). More subtly, the type of scientific information revealed by synthesis was qualitatively different (and of less interest to biologists) than that which might be revealed by cDNA cloning. In other words, the very technique chosen by Genentech reveals important insights into their motivations. Further, the decision to pursue chemical synthesis was made easier by Genentech's willingness to cross interdisciplinary and interinstitutional boundaries. Keiichi Itakura's input as an organic chemist increased as a result of Genentech's focus on expressing a particular hormone, insulin. In sum, Genentech's strategy consisted of a distinct cluster of strategic characteristics which, in concert, increased the team's ability to express insulin in bacteria for the purpose of obtaining a royalty contract with Eli Lilly.

In contrast, the academic researchers' strategies were characterized by the importance of performing experiments that provided novel scientific information or techniques. This focus resulted in the use of cDNA methods by the Harvard and UCSF researchers. While the cDNA method provided scientific focus, this experimental strategy forced the academic researchers to overcome significant regulatory barriers. However, these barriers were not insurmountable except when the research required the use of human genetic material. The choice of cDNA strategies highlights the trade-off between scientific and commercial goals: human genetic material was relatively unnecessary for the scientific agenda, but it was paramount for success in the commercial arena. In conjunction with the focus on nonhuman genetic material, the cDNA strategy leveraged the disciplinary focus of these labs: molecular biology and biochemistry. The synthetic process, while "a quick way to get a result" (telephone interview, W. Rutter, 1993), would have required the input of organic chemists such as Itakura or Khorana. The Gilbert and Rutter-Goodman teams chose the insulin project in order to explore the novel techniques and emerging processes of rDNA research, as this research related to their own discipline. These researchers were not necessarily interested in expressing insulin, per se. Instead, the isolation of the insulin gene and the expression and secretion of insulin in bacteria reflected the discipline-specific priorities of biochemists and molecular biologists. Insulin was studied, not because of its commercial importance, but because it was a "studiable gene" (telephone interview, W. Rutter, 1993). Thus, in contrast with the Genentech strategy, the cluster of characteristics that identify the academic researchers (cDNA cloning, the focus on nonhuman genetic material, and relative disciplinary insularity) reflect the fundamentally different incentives and goals of these researchers.

Interlab Competition

In the previous two subsections, we characterized the incentives and strategies of the three research teams. These characterizations can now be employed to understand the often-cited role of interlab competition in the progress of science and in commercialization. Stephen Hall, among others, views the insulin research as a classic science "race," where different researchers focusing on the same goal attempt to establish experimental precedent for the purpose of scientific prestige and commercial appropriability.[40] In contrast, the evidence seems to suggest a somewhat more subtle and indirect form of competition between these labs. For most of the period studied, the academic researchers and the Genentech researchers were not directly in competition, although the academic researchers were in competition with each other. Only during the summer of 1978, when both the Harvard and UCSF lab chiefs pursued explicit linkages with commercial firms, did the existence of Genentech change the approach and strategies of the academic researchers. Indeed, the existence of divergent goals between the academic and commercial researchers precluded the possibility of a three-way race.

The crucial distinction here is between the competition that existed between the academic teams and the possibility of a race between academic and commercial researchers for the purpose of financial gain. The scientific content of the insulin research dictated that the research would contain competition. In particular, the set of important experimental questions was well-defined and agreed upon by the biochemistry community. For example, successful insertion of the rat insulin gene (performed by the UCSF researchers) was an agreed-upon milestone in recombinant research. Primacy in the achievement of insertion ensured scientific prestige. This type of competition is not *necessarily* wasteful or unproductive, however. Walter Gilbert remarks that "it is hard to do science in isolation . . . the fact that other groups are working on a project validates your own

---

[40]Hall's book is subtitled *The Race to Synthesize a Human Gene.*

research plan" (telephone interview with William Gilbert, Professor, Department of Molecular Biology and Biochemistry, Harvard University, February 18, 1993). Moreover, the existence of clear research goals allows lab chiefs to devote their efforts to successful experimental design rather than the development of research questions. Further, there is strong evidence of this type of competition between the UCSF and Harvard lab groups. William Rutter, in fact, distinguishes between the achievements of Genentech, which he describes as a "chemical challenge, not a biological challenge," and his lab's competition with the Harvard group: "There wasn't a race [for commercial appropriability] . . . but it certainly was a race between Wally Gilbert and myself . . . we were engaged in an intense competition to get that gene" (telephone interview with William Rutter, Professor of Biochemistry, University of California, San Francisco, and President, Chiron Corporation, June 14, 1993). Members of the Harvard group, including Gilbert and Efstratiadis, agree (telephone interview, W. Gilbert, 1993), noting the fundamental similarities in approach between the two academic groups. The chemical synthesis approach pursued by Genentech did not noticeably heighten the level of competition at the labs of the two academic teams.

Bob Swanson at Genentech, in contrast, exploited the competitive nature of his researchers to focus organizational resources on the successful expression of human insulin in bacteria. "Definitely the name Wally Gilbert was in Swanson's mouth all the time. That we had to beat him. But I think Swanson used that as a management tool to keep pressure on Goeddel, knowing that Goeddel was so competitive" (Roberto Crea, quoted in Hall, 1988, p. 219). Ironically, by the time that Gilbert *started* to seriously explore the possibility of expression of human material for commercialization, Genentech had nearly *completed* its mission. Moreover, the Harvard group was at a tremendous disadvantage from the viewpoint of commercialization. The Gilbert team had to conduct experiments under extremely restrictive conditions (P4), their expression system was not designed for the promotion of high yields, and they did not possess a reliable method for "harvesting" the insulin once it was produced by bacteria. In contrast, the Genentech effort, having focused on commercialization from the outset, had systematically overcome these hurdles before the summer of 1978. In sum, to the extent that there was a race for commercialization between Genentech and the Gilbert team, the race was entirely uneven. Genentech's organizational focus provided it with clear advantages over Gilbert's group, which resulted in commercial success and financial appropriability.

Conclusions: Consequences of Insulin Research for Future University-Industry Interactions

The patterns highlighted by this case study must be interpreted cautiously. In particular, the case study approach makes it difficult to distinguish between historical events that are idiosyncratic to the particular situation and the presence of more general trends and behavioral phenomena. This distinction is important here as the insulin experiments and the development of synthetic insulin are landmark events in the history of both biotechnology and biochemistry. The insulin case is "special" as it occurred at a particularly unique juncture within the rDNA revolution and both the scientific and commercial goals were highly focused. Moreover, the insulin research, in conjunction with contemporary research activities,[41] conditioned and guided the development of university-industry interaction within biotechnology. Because of the idiosyncratic nature of the insulin research, the focus of the analysis in this subsection will be upon the set of phenomena in the insulin research that seem to have played a role in the future development of biotechnology and university-industry organization and interaction.

Perhaps the most important lesson to be learned from this case study is that firms and university labs represent fundamentally different organizational structures. Most of the important differences between firms and universities can be understood by examining the differences in their goals. As examined above, university researchers face trade-offs in pursuing the commercialization of basic research results. These trade-offs, by and large, are not present for biotechnology firms (in this case, Genentech). This case study has highlighted various observable consequences of the heterogeneity in incentives. This heterogeneity highlights the following features of the university-industry frontier:

1. **Firms will organize their scientific strategy and recruit their scientific personnel with the intention of focusing their resources on very specific goals.** Genentech's insulin strategy was consistently focused on the goal of appropriability. While the Genentech team was composed of scientists with university research backgrounds, Swanson and Boyer were careful to choose researchers whose goals were aligned with Genentech's: the expression of insulin in bacteria. The evasion of cumbersome regulation, the pursuit of techniques that would provide high protein yield, and the premium on the rapidity of execution (regardless of cost) were all components of Genentech's focused strategy. The university researchers, on the other hand, attempted to exploit the commercial properties of their research in conjunction with the production of important biological information. This resulted in the use of cDNA methods, which re-

---

[41]Some of the more public contemporary work included the human growth hormone research, as well as the highly publicized debate at Harvard University concerning the university's potential exploitation of genetic engineering. Briefly, Harvard proposed that a corporation be set up which would manage the commercial exploitation of technology discovered by Harvard researchers. The proposal, which received extensive national coverage, was abandoned because of opposition from faculty and alumni.

quired compliance with safety regulations, more difficult challenges in potential scale-up, and a longer time horizon for the purpose of commercial production.

2. **University departments will often be "second-place" finishers in competitive, time-dependent innovation**. One of the most important consequences of heterogeneity is the increase in the probability that appropriable rents will, in fact, accrue to firms rather than university labs. While a university lab might eventually be able to focus enough resources to produce appropriable information, a firm will often be able to establish the important commercial result precedentially. Obviously, this is not always true (as innovation success has an important random component). But, given the existence of heterogeneous incentives, it will be true on average. Within the insulin research, Genentech had neared the completion of its initial research program by the time that the Harvard and UCSF researchers had started to seriously organize their commercial activities.

3. **Despite the existence of a strong tradition of scientific purity and commercial disinterest, there existed little difficulty in persuading university basic researchers to attack applied commercial problems. However, the actual transition takes time**. All of the researchers involved in the insulin experiments had been trained in and had operated in noncorporate research environments. Bob Swanson, however, was able to persuade a critical number of researchers (first, and most notably, Herbert Boyer) to attempt commercial problems. However, the development of the Genentech corporate research culture took time to cultivate. Indeed, the somatostatin experiment represents an important transition period for the Genentech researchers as they performed an experiment with little direct commercial value in the context of a corporate funding relationship. The same can be said for the other research teams examined here. Both the Harvard and UCSF researchers developed corporate affiliations by the end of the summer of 1978. While these corporate relationships conditioned future research strategies of these labs, they were of little import in the determination of the strategy for exploring insulin. In an important sense, the Biogen and Lilly funding relationships with the Gilbert and UCSF labs, respectively, needed time to develop before commercially relevant work could be achieved. This transition precluded the ability of these labs to achieve the level of appropriability for their insulin research that Genentech achieved.[42]

4. **There exists a social trade-off between the level of knowledge spillovers and the degree of appropriability. University research is organized around the former, biotechnology firms around the latter**. The desire for appropriability competes with the desire for openness in science and innova-

---

[42]Both the Harvard and UCSF labs received important patents based upon their insulin research. The level of income derived from these patents is small, however, compared to Genentech's exploitation of its insulin success to transform itself into a billion-dollar pharmaceutical company.

tion. The long tradition of openness in university research diminishes the organizational capability of universities to financially capitalize on innovations occurring within their sphere. Firms such as Genentech, in contrast, are created explicitly to ensure the researcher's property rights over innovations.

These four features of the university-industry relationship result from the heterogeneity in incentives and are highlighted in this case study of insulin. Contemporary debate of the insulin research, in fact, explored some of these issues or at least noted the difference between the activities of firms and university labs. Indeed, the emerging biotechnology industry seemed to have grasped some of these features in their subsequent organization of knowledge production and transfer. For example, despite proposals to create university-owned corporations that would manage biotechnology research (e.g., at Harvard), no major university pursued this strategy. Instead, molecular biology and biochemistry departments have become important training sites for industrial researchers as well as serving as a nexus for information dissemination. Moreover, university labs have continued to push forward the boundaries of fundamental scientific knowledge (perhaps best exemplified by the Human Genome Project). Thus, the division of labor that emerged out of the early years of the rDNA revolution resulted, at least partially, from the comparative advantages of industrial and university researchers. Moreover, this organization of labor augmented the possibility for complementary interaction along the university-industry frontier.

ACKNOWLEDGMENTS

This paper was prepared for a conference sponsored by the Institute of Medicine's Committee on Technological Innovation in Medicine. I would like to thank Cathy Fazio, Joshua Gans, Annetine Gelijns, Deval Leshkari and, most especially, Nathan Rosenberg, for their discussions and comments on this work. I would also like to thank the numerous participants in the insulin research who agreed to be interviewed and provided me with their time and thoughtfulness. All errors and omissions, of course, are my own.

REFERENCES

Arora, A., and Gambardella, A. 1989. Complementarity and external linkages: The strategies of large firms in biotechnology. *CEPR Discussion Paper 167*. Stanford, Calif.: Stanford University.

Braithwaite, A., and Smith, F. J. 1985. *Chromatographic Methods*, 4th ed. New York: Chapman and Hall.

Cohen, S. 1982. Gene expression in heterospecific hosts. In: W. Whelan and S. Black, eds. *From Genetic Experimentation to Biotechnology—The Critical Transition*. New York: John Wiley and Sons.

Fudenberg, D., Gilbert, R., Stiglitz, J., and Tirole, J. 1983. Preemption, leapfrogging, and competition in patent races. *European Economic Review* 22:3–31.

Hall, S. S. 1988. *Invisible Frontiers: The Race to Synthesize a Human Gene.* London: Sidgwick & Jackson.

Johnson, J. S. 1983. Human insulin from recombinant DNA technology. *Science* 219(February 11):632–637.

Kenney, M. 1986. *Biotechnology: The University-Industry Complex.* New Haven, Conn.: Yale University Press.

Kolata, G. B. 1976. DNA sequencing: A new era in molecular biology. *Science* 192(May 14):645–647.

Krimsky, S. 1982. *Genetic Alchemy: The Social History of the Recombinant DNA Controversy.* Cambridge, Mass.: MIT Press.

Lewin, R. 1978. Profile of a genetic engineer. *New Scientist* 79(September 28):924–926.

Maugh, T. H. 1976. The artificial gene: It's synthesized and it works in cells. *Science* 194(October 1):44.

McKelvey, M. 1993. *Exploring University-Industry Relations Through the Case of rDNA Human Growth Hormone.* Unpublished manuscript. Sweden: University of Linkoping.

Morrow, J., Cohen, S., Chang, A., et al. 1974. Replication and transcription of eukaryotic DNA in *Escherichia coli. Proceedings of the National Academy of Sciences, USA* 71(May):1743–1747.

Rosenberg, N. 1992. Scientific instrumentation and university research. *Research Policy* 21:381–390.

Sylvester, E., and Klotz, L. 1983. *The Gene Age.* New York: Scribner's.

Ullrich, A., Shine, J., Chirgwin, J., et al. 1977. Rat insulin genes: Construction of plasmids containing the coding sequences. *Science* 196(June 17):1313–1319.

Villa-Komaroff, L., Efstratiadis, A., Broome, S., et al. 1978. A bacterial clone synthesizing proinsulin. *Proceedings of the National Academy of Sciences, USA* 75(August):3727–3731.

Wade, N. 1977. Recombinant DNA: NIH rules broken in insulin gene project. *Science* 197(September 30):1342.

Watson, J. 1968. *The Double Helix.* New York: Atheneum Press.

Watson, J. 1976. *Molecular Biology of the Gene,* 3rd ed. Menlo Park, Calif.: W. A. Benjamin.

8

The Division of Innovative Labor in Biotechnology

ASHISH ARORA AND ALFONSO GAMBARDELLA

The growing use of general and abstract knowledge, based upon an increasing understanding of principles governing phenomena and the tremendous growth in computational capabilities, has opened up new possibilities for specialization (Arora and Gambardella, 1992). The breadth of downstream applications of abstract principles and the feasibility of representing them in a universal and codified form implies that information can be divided into "pieces" that can be usefully recomposed together to form "larger pieces" of information, provided a general and comprehensive framework for integrating the information exists. With suitable contracts, the individual pieces of information and knowledge can be bought and sold. This lays the basis for economic agents to specialize according to comparative advantage, thereby giving rise to the division of inventive labor.

A number of authors have commented upon the growing importance of networks and strategic alliances in innovation (see, for example, Mowery, 1988). Some have gone so far as to argue that it is now difficult to identify the innovator with a particular organization. Imai (1988), *inter alia*, has suggested that the locus of innovation is shifting from the individual firm to a network of firms, where the network itself is the innovating institution. Instead, we submit that networks and strategic alliances are best viewed as important special cases of the more general phenomenon of a division of innovative labor.

To highlight the use of general and abstract knowledge in innovation, we focus here upon one sector of the increasingly diverse "biotechnology industry," the human diagnostics and therapeutics sector, often referred to as "biopharmaceuticals" (Burrill, 1989). Biotechnology is an example *par excellence* of the use of general and abstract knowledge in innovation. Technological advances based on genetic engineering and molecular biology have deeply affected the pharmaceutical industry. They have given great impetus to the possibility of understanding the "causes" of diseases and the action of drugs. Reliance upon random screening of compounds to find what may work is giving way to more selective and carefully structured experiments, guided by basic theory. As a result, now researchers can often design drugs on computers and "build" them in labs before extensive experimentation on animals and human beings.[1]

The biotechnology sector also provides a prototypical example of the changing patterns of specialization in inventive activity that we call the division of innovative labor. Historically, large pharmaceutical companies, which integrated activities from research to distribution, have been the primary source of innovation in the industry. The rise of biotechnology, along with a number of related economic forces, has made possible, and to a large extent forced, specialization and cooperation among large pharmaceutical firms and small, research-intensive, biotechnology enterprises. In this network of innovators, universities and research institutions occupy an important place as well.

The next section describes more fully the participants in the division of labor in biotechnology. The section following that discussion examines the different strategies of external linkages from the viewpoint of the large corporations and characterizes the relationship between these different strategies. We then analyze the factors that determine the value that a firm can derive from its external linkages, and the light that throws upon the nature of division of innovative labor. The penultimate section discusses whether the division of innovative labor is socially desirable and the final section provides our conclusion.

PARTICIPANTS IN THE DIVISION OF INNOVATIVE LABOR IN BIOTECHNOLOGY

Up to the 1980s, most new drugs stemmed from systematic investments in internal research and development (R&D) by large corporations (Thomas, 1988). Biotechnology has a "science-push" origin. The initial breakthroughs include the discovery of the double-helix structure of DNA in 1953 and the discovery of the new techniques of recombinant DNA (rDNA) and cell fusion (monoclonal antibodies) in the 1970s, all of which resulted from scientific research within the university system. In addition, there have been significant advances in molecular biology and related fields, such as computer imaging of molecules, which have greatly increased the understanding of the links between molecular structure and

---

[1]We use biotechnology as a convenient short hand for the entire gamut of scientific and technological advances, including recombinant DNA techniques, hybridoma and PCR techniques, and the more fundamental advances in molecular biology, molecular genetics, and biochemistry.

function (and dysfunction). The increased knowledge about the structure of biological molecules such as enzymes and the isolation and cloning of human genes offer new opportunities to develop drugs that can counteract diseases (Gambardella, 1995; Office of Technology Assessment, 1984; Pisano et al., 1988). For instance, the synthesis of the nucleic acid sequence, originally performed at the City of Hope Medical Center, led to the large scale production of rDNA insulin. This was developed, produced, and commercialized by a joint venture between Genentech and Eli Lilly.

Biotechnology, with its strong grounding in basic science, has changed markedly the organizational pattern of the innovation process in this industry. Three types of agents now contribute to the generation, development, and commercialization of new biotechnology products, and particularly of biopharmaceuticals: the universities; small/medium-sized research-intensive firms or the so-called new biotechnology firms (NBFs); and the large "established" chemical and pharmaceutical manufacturers. Many new drugs and therapies now stem from systematic interactions and cooperation between these three types of agents.

Universities and NBFs were important sources of new techniques and products at the outset, and remain very important sources of basic and applied scientific knowledge in this field. However, while collaborations with universities have been common in the pharmaceutical industry for many years (see, for instance, Swann, 1988; Thackeray, 1982), and biotechnology has only intensified an already existing pattern of relationships, the rise of the NBFs is an entirely new phenomenon. Most NBFs were founded during the early 1980s. Their major asset consists of knowledge, especially that embodied in their researchers (Kenney, 1986; Office of Technology Assessment, 1984; Pisano et al., 1988). In many instances they were founded to exploit a discovery made by an individual or group, and they were created by professors or groups of academic scientists. Over a thousand NBFs have been founded in the past decade. Even in a "bad" year such as 1988, some 36 new NBFs were formed (Burrill, 1990).

As Table 8-1 shows, a majority of NBFs are U.S. based. A number of reasons can be cited for the formation of NBFs, and particularly for the finding that a majority are U.S. based. Clearly, their growth was triggered by the rise of new scientific and technological opportunities and the fact that established corporations were late to enter into biotechnology research (see, *inter alia*, Pisano et al., 1988). However, economic forces at work in the U.S. system have played an important role as well. The relationship between universities and industry in this country is unusually close; and there is an availability of finance especially suited for high-risk technology businesses (venture capital and the like; see Florida and Kenney, 1990; Office of Technology Assessment, 1984). The biotech industry in the United States has also benefited considerably from the output of federally sponsored research in this field—often a new product or a method that can rapidly translate into new product opportunities. That is, federally supported research has helped produce discoveries that have, in turn, paved the way to new

TABLE 8-1 Composition of the Biotechnology Industry

Country	Small	Medium	Large
Japan	1	4	46
United States	138	84	65
Europe	39	18	33
Other	21	15	11

NOTE: Small = up to 50 employees; medium = 51–299 employees; large = ≥300 employees.

SOURCE: The table is based upon Chang (1992, p. 15, Table 1). It covers all companies listed in Bioscan (April 1991) that are involved in human diagnostics or human therapeutics and that provide information on employment.

business opportunities. These opportunities have been exploited by the institutions performing the research, by NBFs through their academic ties, or by NBFs or other companies taking advantage of the knowledge generated by public research. Finally, the United States has followed an aggressive policy of defining and strengthening intellectual property rights. In this context, the landmark 1980 Supreme Court decision of *Diamond* v. *Chakrabarty*, which established the legality of patenting of life forms, is frequently cited as providing the security needed by small, research-intensive biotech firms whose major asset is their research capability.

The basic assets of NBFs are skills and know-how relating to applied laboratory research. Their close ties to the academic system, their collegial atmosphere, and the possibility of using incentive-based compensation schemes (such as stock options for researchers) have given them a comparative advantage in research.[2] A typical product of an NBF could be a new protein, obtained from genetically engineered organisms, that can be potentially used for diagnostic or therapeutic purposes.

The synthesis of a new protein, however, while an important step, does not exhaust the entire innovation cycle. In pharmaceuticals, downstream development of compounds is a long and costly process, in no small measure due to the stringent regulation of clinical tests. Most NBFs lack the organizational and financial resources for undertaking such developments; nor do they have adequate commercialization capabilities (Burrill, 1989; Kenney, 1986). Furthermore, venture capitalists backing NBFs often press for relatively short-term cash

---

[2]Lerner (1991) provides evidence (measured by citations to scientific publications) that the patents of NBFs are more strongly based in science than the patents of a matched sample of large firms active in biotechnology.

returns, which are incompatible with the long time cycles of pharmaceutical innovation. As a result, many NBFs end up offering their skills or potential new products to larger firms for research collaborations and joint product developments instead of undertaking development, manufacturing, and commercialization on their own.[3]

Large established chemical and pharmaceutical companies have the engineering know-how required to scale up from the laboratory bench to large-scale manufacturing, and further to control the industrial-scale processes. More importantly, they have the financial capabilities for conducting long and costly clinical trials. They are familiar with clinical testing procedures and the regulatory process, and they have established commercialization networks.[4]

A number of other factors have raised the incentives of the large firms to take advantage of the specialized expertise and product opportunities offered by the NBFs (see Grabowski, 1991, and Telling, 1992). U.S. policy on generic drugs in the 1980s (and particularly the Waxman-Hatch Act in 1984) reduced substantially the property rights of the pharmaceutical companies in their main products when patents expire. As a result, all major drug manufacturers had to undertake significant efforts to create a new portfolio of patented products. In addition, the evolution of the market from one where doctors order medicines without much attention to cost toward more conscious, expert buyers has required that products be not only new, but also superior.

Large firms have, then, found resorting to NBFs for new product ideas useful for several reasons. First, as suggested earlier, the research of the NBFs is often partly subsidized by investor capital and possibly public money via university linkages. Second, royalty payments to NBFs are, in most cases, contingent on success. Finally, because biotech firms are typically pressed for cash, large companies can negotiate favorable terms. In other words, an alliance with an NBF can be beneficial to a large firm because it does not require a large financial commitment, and because it allows the large firm useful access to knowledge that has in part been supported by public funds and in part by the investing public.[5]

In sum, because large firms and NBFs control assets that are largely complementary, systematic collaborations between them have arisen. Moreover, as we saw, economic forces have reinforced this trend by pushing both the NBFs to take advantage of the downstream capabilities of large firms, and the large firms to avail themselves of the upstream research skills of the NBFs.

---

[3]The total turnover of many NBFs is, indeed, still composed for the most part of research contracts to larger firms rather than actual product sales. See, for instance, Burrill (1989).

[4]They also have the financial and organizational capabilities for conducting research based upon "lumpy" assets (e.g., molecular design based on expensive supercomputers). In this case, large firms can offer complementary expertise in more "upstream" research as well.

[5]We would like to thank Gerald Laubach for a very useful and enlightening discussion of these points.

Universities also control assets and skills that are to some extent complementary to those of both the NBFs and the large firms (typically, upstream scientific capabilities). As a result, the growth of the industry has hinged upon network-like relationships based upon extensive collaborations and a division of labor between these three types of agents.[6]

COLLABORATION STRATEGIES OF LARGE FIRMS

There are a number of different types of external linkages that large firms have used. Following the literature on this topic, one can identify four main types of linkages that large firms have formed with other agents in biotechnology:[7] (1) they enter into research and/or joint development agreements with other firms; (2) they form research agreements with universities; (3) they invest in the capital stock of NBFs (minority participation); (4) they acquire NBFs. To a large extent, each of these four strategies enables the firm to gain access to a particular set of tangible or intangible resources necessary for innovation.[8]

Most agreements signed by large chemical and pharmaceutical producers with other companies tend to be project specific. These agreements, usually with NBFs, focus on "downstream" activities of the innovation cycle. They are aimed at developing and commercializing a particular discovery of the NBF (e.g., the synthesis of a new enzyme or hormone or growth factor) in the areas of specialty chemicals, agricultural biotechnology and, above all, pharmaceuticals.

The agreements with universities tend to focus on more basic research objectives. Large firms finance research activities performed by academic laboratories to acquire, by interacting with university scientists, some familiarity with the basic knowledge in this field. Such agreements, between large firms and universities, are important sources of recruiting qualified scientists and researchers, and also serve as a means by which firms can engage the services of top researchers while these researchers continue to work in environments they find most congenial.[9] Other than these general and "intangible" gains, the agreements with uni-

---

[6]Clearly, there is some overlap between the skills, competencies, and activities of universities, NBFs, and large firms. Many large corporations perform in-house basic and applied research. Universities often perform a good deal of applied research. Many NBFs have in-house basic research skills, and a few others now possess downstream capabilities. Nonetheless, our schematic distinction has an important element of truth and serves well as a first approximation. We shall return below to a fuller discussion of the nature of these comparative advantages.

[7]See, for instance, Daly (1985), Kenney (1986), Office of Technology Assessment (1984), and Pisano et al. (1988).

[8]The following discussion on the different forms of external linkages of the large firms in biotechnology draws upon Arora and Gambardella (1990).

[9]Kenney (1986) suggests that a "preferential access" to trained manpower is an important reason for university–corporate linkages in biotechnology.

versities also serve a more explicit objective of the large firms. Given the short distance between science and commercialization in biotechnology, an agreement with a university can provide the large firm with the option of licensing any new discovery of that research center (within the scope defined by the agreement). This is an advantage for a firm that can rapidly translate those new discoveries into commercializable products.

Minority participation in the capital stock of small biotech start-up firms is a means of monitoring the internal research activities of the NBFs. By acquiring part of the capital stock of an NBF, the large companies may also hope to establish a "preferential" linkage with that company, which may be useful to preempt rivals in the commercialization of relevant discoveries made by the NBF. Moreover, in keeping with the theoretical predictions of Williamson (1985), such investments may be useful in averting problems of moral hazard by serving as tokens of good faith. In 1986, for instance, American Home Products bought 13.5 percent of the shares of California Biotechnology, and in that same year the two companies entered into formal arrangements in the fields of cardiovascular drugs, veterinary therapeutics, and drug delivery systems. Other examples of this sort include the cases of Abbott and Amgen, American Cyanamid and Cytogen, Johnson & Johnson and Cytogen, and SmithKline-Beecham and Amgen. Similarly, British Biotechnology obtained its start-up capital in 1986 from a consortium that included SmithKline Beecham, and later the two entered into a joint venture for a line of anti-arthritic therapies based upon matrix metallo-proteinex inhibitors developed by British Biotechnology.

As far as acquisitions are concerned, there seem to exist two different—and somewhat contrary—motives for acquiring a small biotech company. On the one hand, large companies that have substantial in-house capabilities, longer experience in biotechnology, and more active involvement in the field aim at acquiring NBFs specialized in particular areas of biotechnology research. The experience and in-house expertise of the large companies enables them to evaluate more accurately the likely contributions of the set of specialized resources that are being acquired. On the other hand, the direct acquisition of a biotechnology firm may also represent a way of "catching up" for late entrants.[10]

These remarks suggest that each of the four types of external linkages targets a separate goal of the large firms, and thus they are mutually complementary.

---

[10]Compare the acquisitions in 1986 of Hybritech by Eli Lilly and of Genetics System and Oncogen by Bristol Myers. Eli Lilly is one of the most research-intensive pharmaceutical companies worldwide, and was an early entrant in biotechnology research. It sought to complement its generalized expertise in biotechnology with know-how in monoclonal antibodies, wherein Hybritech had specialized capabilities. Bristol-Myers has strong marketing capabilities, but it is less research-intensive. Through acquisitions, it sought generalized expertise in the new area of biotechnology. See Gambardella (1992 and 1995).

Through agreements with other firms (particularly with NBFs), the large firms can develop and commercialize new biotech products after the NBFs have undertaken the initial upstream stages. The agreements with universities provide the large firms with access to basic scientific knowledge. Minority participation enables them to acquire familiarity with the internal research activities of the NBF. Acquisitions add specialized or generalized internal knowledge to the large firms in some areas of the biotech business.

In Arora and Gambardella (1990), we presented a formal model of the complementarity hypothesis and also tested for complementarity between the four kinds of external linkages for a sample of 81 large U.S., European, and Japanese chemical and pharmaceutical companies, during 1983–1989. Our empirical results support the idea that the four strategies are mutually complementary. We found that firms that tended to have a large number of one type of linkage also tended to have a greater number of the others. This suggests that the (marginal) "value" of each of the four strategies is greater the larger the number of the other types of linkages undertaken by the firm.[11] *In other words, firms differ more in the extent to which they seek out external linkages, rather than in the specific types of linkages that they do seek.*

EVALUATING AND USING TECHNOLOGICAL INFORMATION

These findings raise the question: What factors determine the payoff from external linkages? We offer a different perspective from that of traditional analyses, which have been framed largely in terms of transaction-cost economics. The transaction-cost perspective would suggest that firms attempt to internalize the knowledge-based assets required for innovation. Hence, firms with strong in-house research capabilities would be less likely to enter into strategic alliances.

Pisano (1990) has provided the strongest case for this perspective in the context of biotechnology. Pisano's results are based upon a sample of some 92 biotech projects, at the preclinical and earlier stage, from 30 large pharmaceutical firms. He found that the smaller the number of NBFs active in a particular therapeutic area, the greater the number of previous projects the large firm had carried out (through in-house efforts alone) in that particular therapeutic area; and, possibly, the greater the fraction of their sales accounted for by pharmaceuticals, the more likely the pharmaceutical firms were to perform the R&D exclusively in house. The interpretation of these results is that where small numbers of NBFs are bargaining and in-house capability is great, internalization of projects is favored so as to economize on transaction costs.

But Pisano's empirical evidence is amenable to alternative interpretations.

---

[11]We also found that, for these large firms, size or nationality did not affect their propensity to engage in external linkages and had relatively low explanatory power.

The smaller the number of NBFs in a particular area, the less likely it is that the large firm would be able to find a suitable partner with the appropriate research capabilities. Moreover, Pisano assumes that the choice or problem facing the large firm can be adequately represented by assuming that the project is initiated by the large firm, which then decides whether to use external subcontractors or not. Our understanding of the industry is that NBFs initate the bulk of the new projects in the sector, some of which may be offered to large firms for their participation.

Furthermore, firms such as Eli Lilly, Johnson & Johnson, and Monsanto, which began their in-house research efforts early (in some cases even before the start of the 1980s), were precisely the firms that led in making external collaborative alliances. In essence, the analogy with the make-or-buy decision in production can be misleading in the context of innovation. To be sure, transaction costs are important, but technological knowledge is a special type of good. It requires a great deal of specialized knowledge and skill to successfully utilize technological information. In order to "buy" such knowledge, one has to have a great deal of prior knowledge—inexperienced and unskilled buyers are at a severe disadvantage.

In other words, it is precisely firms with strong in-house R&D capabilities that would derive the greatest value from external linkages. Cohen and Levinthal (1989) argue that firms invest in R&D for two purposes. On the one hand, they invest in R&D to generate innovations; on the other hand, R&D serves as a device for exploiting external research. Rosenberg (1990) argues that in-house basic research is necessary to monitor the flow of scientific information in the outside world. Mowery (1981) showed that, during 1921–1945, large U.S. firms, when starting new innovation projects, also contracted out part of the research to specialized institutes. These studies emphasize the potential synergies between external and internal knowledge. However, their discussion does not deal with the multidimensionality of knowledge, and therefore does not "unpackage" the source of the synergies.

In Arora and Gambardella (1994b), we attempted to distinguish between two types of knowledge-based capabilities: The *ability to utilize* and the *ability to evaluate* information. In the present context, therefore, there are two considerations involved in entering into an external alliance. The first is concerned with the skills and competencies that the large firm has in the development and commercialization of the innovation—in other words, how capable the large firm is of utilizing the information that it is "purchasing" from an NBF. The second consideration is related but logically distinct and has to do with the ability of the firm to form judgments about the potential usefulness of the information that it is buying.

Consider, therefore, a large corporation at the point of deciding whether or not to enter into a collaborative agreement with an NBF. The latter typically offers an "idea." For instance, it may have synthesized in an *E. coli* culture a protein that is closely related to some physiological disorder; or it may have discovered a way of inducing a gene to express itself. In some instances, the NBF may offer a useful technique relating, for example, to a way of separating a particular protein from other products produced by a cell culture or a delivery system. The large firm funds any further research that may be needed, and then may "license-in" the idea for further development. One can think of each such link as the purchase of an option on a "project." The initial investment made in a typical external agreement is not very large relative to the total R&D budgets of these corporations. Typical sums involved in these linkages are on the order of (at most) 5–10 percent of the total expenditure involved in introducing a drug.

The willingness of a firm to invest in such a linkage will depend first and foremost on whether it has the requisite development competencies in the particular therapeutic area, and on whether it has *underutilized* downstream capabilities for successful commercialization.[12] A slightly different way of putting it is to note that firms' commercialization capabilities are fixed in the short run and are to some extent specific to particular therapeutic areas. The firm would like to be able to utilize its commercialization capabilities to the fullest extent possible. It follows, therefore, that the better (and more extensive) these downstream capabilities of commercialization (or, as we put it, the better the ability to utilize), the greater the willingness of the large firm to invest in an external alliance.

However, the willingness to invest also depends upon the firm's ability to evaluate the likely commercial value of the project. Here the relationship is rather subtle. Since the investment is tantamount to the purchase of an option, firms that are better able to forecast the value of the project will be more discerning in their external collaborations. They are able to focus upon the more promising linkages.

In Arora and Gambardella (1994b) we formally show that the two kinds of knowledge-based capabilities have rather different empirical predictions for the propensity of the firm to engage in such linkages. The better the ability to utilize, the greater, on average, the number of external linkages; on the other hand, all else held equal, the better the ability to evaluate, the fewer the number of external linkages (but these are of greater expected value).

How does one empirically distinguish between the two types of abilities? The measures one chooses have to be rooted in the specificities of the industrial sector in question. In our study, based on a sample of the 26 largest U.S. pharmaceutical companies, we used two variables as measures of the ability to utilize. The first variable was the ratio of R&D expenditures to sales. Since these are large corporations, one would expect a research-intensive firm to also have in

---

[12]Gerald Laubach has emphasized to us the importance of replenishing product pipelines. Firms that have strong abilities to utilize and to evaluate, such as Merck, may nonetheless not have many external alliances if their product pipelines are relatively full.

place other assets, such as a marketing and distribution network, that are necessary for successful commercialization of research outcomes. In other words, R&D intensity can serve as a proxy for a "package" of research capabilities and complementary downstream assets. The second variable is the stock of biotechnology patents applied for in the United States. This variable is intended to capture the extent to which a firm has invested in biotechnology-related research in the past years, and therefore its ability to utilize external technological information in that area.[13]

What publicly available measure can one use for the ability to evaluate? It has been argued that science provides information that helps restrict the search for successful innovations at the downstream, applied R&D stages. Superior scientific capabilities enable the firm to reduce the uncertainty about the outcome of an individual project (David et al., 1988; Nelson, 1961). As noted earlier, Rosenberg (1990) has argued that in-house basic research is useful primarily for being "plugged in" to external information flows. Since a great deal of relevant information in biotechnology is science based, an in-house scientific capability is crucial for evaluating and assessing information originating outside of the firm's boundaries.[14] As a measure of in-house scientific capabilities, we used the average number of scientific papers (stock) published by the personnel of the firms divided by total sales.[15]

In our empirical tests, we found that these measures performed well. The measures of the ability to utilize information are positively related to the number of external linkages, and the measure for scientific capability is negatively related to the number of linkages.[16] These results also help us clarify an important point. Our discussion might have unintentionally suggested that within the division of innovative labor in the biotech industry, research is performed by NBFs, while large firms provide only downstream capabilities. This is not true. Large firms perform a great deal of upstream research. In fact, our results suggest that

---

[13]The use of patents as a measure of the technological strength of pharmaceutical firms is supported by the results reported in Narin et al. (1987).

[14]It should be noted that by "science" we mean abstract knowledge and representations in terms of general and universal categories. The use of such abstraction allows the researcher to delineate and characterize more carefully the set of possible outcomes, eliminate a number of other possibilities, and hence be able to focus upon a smaller set of more carefully designed experiments. Furthermore, information from diverse sources can be better integrated to throw light upon the problem at hand and thereby allow a more informed and accurate judgment about the likelihood of the success of the project. See Arora and Gambardella (1994a and 1992) for further discussion and references.

[15]Halperin and Chakrabarti (1987) found that company scientific publications are highly correlated with the number of elite researchers employed by the firm (more so than patenting by the firms).

[16]In Arora and Gambardella (1994b) we focused only on the agreements of large firms with NBFs, and neglected minority participation and acquisitions. We also examined the agreements with universities and other research institutions. However, alliances with universities did not appear to be related in the same way to the measures, suggesting that alliances with universities are more properly thought of as providing access to knowledge and as a means of building up in-house competencies.

internal research provides the necessary knowledge to extract greater rents from alliances. In-house capabilities of a more fundamental nature help in directing external investments toward those alliances with greater potential payoff.[17]

THE DIVISION OF INNOVATIVE LABOR:
TRANSIENT AND UNDESIRABLE?

Our results bear upon another important question regarding the biotechnology sector as well. As widely discussed among economists, managers, and analysts, an important question about the future of the biotech industry (and more generally of the pharmaceutical industry) is whether the new division of innovative labor is merely a transient phenomenon. We saw that transaction-cost perspectives lead to the view that once large firms acquire sufficient knowledge, they will tend to withdraw from external linkages and revert to in-house R&D alone. The available evidence is mixed, but on the whole it supports the idea that while the patterns of specialization and division of labor have changed over time, no clear trend towards extensive internalization and integration exists.[18]

Moreover, we submit that a modest decline in the number of alliances between large firms and NBFs is not inconsistent with the division of innovative labor. Instead it reflects greater learning about external linkages on the part of agents involved. Market forces are increasingly selecting the NBFs not only according to their ability to perform "good science," but also according to their ability to translate science into commercializable outcomes. Thus, fewer NBFs survive as more than transient start-up "gamblers," which has a negative scale effect on the number of alliances. More importantly, large firms, and especially the most innovative ones, have now become sufficiently familiar with the knowledge base of biotechnology, and particularly with its upstream scientific base. As the results discussed in the previous section would suggest, firms have therefore become more discerning in their choice of partners, and hence form fewer but potentially more valuable alliances.

A final question is whether a division of innovative labor in biotechnology is socially desirable. Florida and Kenney (1990), *inter alia*, see the emergence of NBFs as socially undesirable. They claim that venture capital funding leads to a

---

[17]Max Link, the CEO of Sandoz Pharma Ltd., epitomized this view: "We believe that the stronger a multinational is in a particular field, the higher the probability that a cooperation will yield positive results" (*Scrip*, 1991).

[18]Some recent reports about the industry suggest a moderate decline in the number of alliances between large firms and NBFs (Burrill and Lee, 1991). On the other hand, Barabanti et al. (1992) find an increase in the total number of collaborations of 21 major pharmaceutical companies in biotechnology, as well as in the average number of collaborations per firm, in these three periods: up to 1983, 1984–1987, 1988–1991. Their results also indicate considerable volatility in the patterns of collaborative alliances.

demand for quick and high returns, which leads to a short-term focus and myopic decisionmaking. Moreover, in their view, the formation of a large number of NBFs causes a "fragmentation" of capabilities by spreading the available scientific and technological expertise too thinly. Furthermore, the "patent race" nature of NBFs suggests a misallocation of resources, with too many NBFs operating in the same niche. Hence they expect a decline in the comparative advantage of NBFs, with a given NBF losing its "innovativeness," as well as NBFs of later vintage being less innovative than their predecessors.[19] Implicitly, therefore, Florida and Kenney are of the view that the beneficial advantages of specialization and division of labor are outweighed by the costs of information exchange and integration, as well as the destructive competition for resources and markets that may accompany a division of labor.[20]

While a division of labor in innovation can, in fact, produce dispersion of capabilities, with implied high coordination costs, it is also true that fragmentation of capabilities is a more serious problem in instances where the knowledge base for innovation is tacit and context-specific. When the knowledge base is tacit and context-dependent, it is difficult to exchange technological information across organizational boundaries.

As we have argued, effective information exchange has become easier. Increased understanding of scientific and technological principles, coupled with the use of computer-based models, makes it possible to generate and utilize information that is expressed in relatively general and abstract forms: that is, in forms that are common to different organizations and that can be applied to different contexts. This increased universality in the form of information eases information exchange for innovation, and encourages specialization and division of labor according to comparative advantage.[21]

Biotechnology exemplifies the increasing use of general and abstract knowledge for innovation, and the consequent possibilities that have arisen for a new division of labor in inventive activity. This perspective leads us to suspect that the division of labor in biotechnology will prove to be more enduring than traditional Chandlerian or transaction-cost perspectives would suggest.

The social desirability of a division of innovative labor in general arises in part from the differences in comparative advantages that depend upon the size and nature of different organizational forms. As many authors have argued, large

---

[19]However, Lerner (1991) finds no evidence to suggest that the research productivity of NBFs (as measured by citation-weighted patents) in his sample declines over time. Lerner also reports that the research productivity of NBFs in his sample is significantly higher than that of the matched sample of large companies.

[20]It is interesting to note that Merges and Nelson (1990) take the opposite view regarding the desirability of a large number of start-ups. They argue that, from an evolutionary perspective, diversity is likely to promote the rate of growth.

[21]We spell out this argument more fully in Arora and Gambardella (1994a) where we relate it to the feasibility and social desirability of a division of innovative labor more generally.

and small firms have "natural" comparative advantages in different stages of innovation (see, for example, Arrow, 1962). Smaller firms have flexible and informal organizational structures, which facilitate inventiveness. As Arrow suggests, the organizational distance between inventors and the people making decisions on the internal allocation of resources to innovation projects is greater in larger firms. The greater distance creates loss of information in communication and greater asymmetry of information. Smaller companies are, therefore, better able to undertake more novel (and riskier) projects, provided they can finance such projects. In contrast, larger firms have superior organizational and financial capabilities (including easier access to financial markets because of information asymmetries and the like) for large-scale development, production, and marketing.

Consistent with our analysis of comparative advantage, NBFs have found "go-it-alone" strategies easier in the less lucrative market for diagnostic kits, especially in-vitro kits, because the development and regulatory procedures are simpler. Even in such markets, however, complementary assets such as the ability to supply diagnostic equipment and previous experience in dealing with hospitals have proved to be of great importance for established companies such as Abbott. Lacking these complementary assets for commercialization, NBFs such as Hybritech and Genetic Systems were forced to sell out, to Eli Lilly and Bristol-Myers, respectively. (See also Arora and Gambardella, 1990; Barabanti et al., 1992; and Orsenigo, 1989.) Indeed, most NBFs have found the transition from research to production and marketing a difficult one, and the research orientation of their founders and top management have frequently made it more so.

Perhaps recognizing their comparative advantage, some NBFs have adopted the strategy articulated by Benzon Pharma, a small Danish drug company with a number of alliances with larger firms such as SmithKline Beecham and Schering-Plough. Benzon's strategy is to work on new scientific areas that are applicable to many kinds of drugs. All projects are carried out with the possibility of linking them to the programs of other, usually much larger, pharmaceutical companies (*Financial Times*, 1990). Only a few NBFs like Amgen and Biogen have successfully acquired the complementary assets for commercialization, the former with erythropoietin and colony stimulating factors, and the latter with the interferons.

Even where NBFs have been able to acquire some downstream capabilities, they remain extremely vulnerable to adverse Food and Drug Administration (FDA) findings and other "misfortunes" in production or marketing. The tissue plasminogen activator (t-PA) disappointment led to the acquisition of 60 percent of the capital of Genentech by Hoffman La Roche.[22] Similar problems led to the

---

[22]Interestingly enough, Hoffman La Roche preserved in substantial ways Genentech's autonomy as an independent company, suggesting that this acquisition is more a match of complementary assets than a prototypical case of vertical integration.

merger of Cetus, one of the earliest biotech firms, with Chiron, another "large" NBF. Finally, the value of Centocor's stock dropped by 25 percent after the FDA questioned data on its new septic shock drug. Thereafter, Centocor signed an agreement with Eli Lilly, which hopes to use its expertise in development and FDA regulation, as well as its commercialization capabilities, to revamp Centocor's compound.[23]

A very important question, suggested by the conceptualization of the process as one of division of labor, and one that has not yet been asked in the literature, has to do with the creative destruction of competencies implicit in the downward integration of NBFs. Given that some of the most innovative NBFs, such as Amgen and Biogen, are converting themselves into full-fledged pharmaceutical companies, it would be useful to ask whether the process is inevitable and (a related question) whether it is socially efficient. In other words, even if private incentives point toward integration, one must ask whether these represent the benefits that authors such as Florida and Kenney have pointed toward, or whether these are responses to market imperfections that are widely known but whose ramifications may not be well understood. The answer to the question will have important implications for policy. For instance, strengthening the definition and enforcement of intellectual property rights may slow down or even stop the process of downward integration. At this stage we shall pose it as an important and interesting question for further research.

SUMMARY AND CONCLUSIONS

In this essay we have examined the changing patterns of collaborative alliances in biotechnology. Based on some previous studies on the topic, we discussed how innovation in biotechnology is the outcome of systematic interactions between universities, NBFs, and large pharmaceutical firms. We characterized the different strategies of external linkages from the viewpoint of large firms, and found that they were mutually complementary in that they target distinct but synergistic objectives of the firm. The division of innovative labor that we have studied is taking place in the context of a noticeable increase in the use of general and abstract knowledge in innovation. The breadth of applicability of universal principles offers the possibility of subdivision of the innovation process

---

[23]In this context, it is interesting to note that, while Centocor and the other biotech firms mentioned above seek partnerships for resources and expertise downstream, Eli Lilly is moving in the other direction. It has recently taken serious steps to combat its "not invented here" syndrome. As explicitly declared by its top managers, Lilly seeks extensive alliances with partners that can supply new ideas and products to be pumped into its pipeline. In the early 1990s, Lilly signed a number of such alliances with small/medium research-intensive companies in fields such as molecular design of drugs (Agouron), serotonin-based drugs (Synoptic Pharma), and trauma infections (*Business Week*, 1992).

by allowing "pieces" of technological information to be recombined in a useful and cost-effective manner. However, for a "market" in technology to function effectively, institutions relating to intellectual property, as well as institutions for financing start-up ventures, have to adapt. We argued that "buying" technological information requires a great deal of prior competence and capabilities, very similar to those required for generating new technological information. The nature of the "market" for information and its functioning, and their implications for the organization and rate and direction of innovation, are not fully understood and remain important areas of future research.

ACKNOWLEDGMENTS

We would like to thank Rebecca Henderson and the other participants at the Institute of Medicine workshop, "The University-Industry Interface and Medical Innovation," for comments and discussion. We are especially grateful to Gerald Laubach for detailed comments that were very helpful. All errors are ours.

REFERENCES

Arora, A., and Gambardella, A. 1990. Complementarities and external linkages: The strategies of the large firms in biotechnology. *Journal of Industrial Economics* 37:361–379.

Arora, A., and Gambardella, A. 1992. New trends in technological change. *Rivista Internazionale di Scienze Sociali* 3(July–September):259–277.

Arora, A., and Gambardella, A. 1994a. Changing technology of technological change. *Research Policy* 23:523–532.

Arora, A., and Gambardella, A. 1994b. Evaluating scientific information and utilizing it: Scientific knowledge, technological capability, and external linkages in biotechnology. *Journal of Economic Behavior and Organization* 24:91–114.

Arrow, K. 1962. Economic welfare and the allocation of resources for invention. In: *The Rate and Direction of Inventive Activity*. Princeton, N.J.: Princeton University Press.

Barabanti, P., Gambardella, A., and Orsenigo, L. 1992. The evolution of the forms of collaboration in biotechnology. Unpublished manuscript. Milan: Bocconi University.

Bioscan. 1991. *The Biotechnology Corporate Directory Service* (April). Phoenix, Ariz.: Oryx Press.

Burrill, G. S. 1989. *Biotech 89: Commercialization.* New York: Mary Ann Liebert, Inc.

Burrill, G. S. 1990. *Biotech 90: Into the Next Decade.* New York: Mary Ann Liebert, Inc.

Burrill, G. S., and Lee, K. B. 1991. *Biotech '92: Promise to Reality.* New York: Mary Ann Liebert, Inc.

Business Week. 1992. Lilly looks for a shot of adrenalin. Nov. 23, pp. 70–72.

Chang, L. 1992. Biotechnology and the organization of innovation. Unpublished manuscript. Stanford, Calif.: Department of Economics, Stanford University.

Cohen, W., and Levinthal, D. 1989. Innovation and learning: The two faces of R&D.
    Economic Journal 99(September):569–596.

Daly, P. 1985. *The Biotechnology Business.* London: Francis Pinter.

David, P., Mowery, D., and Steinmueller, E. 1988. The economic analysis of payoffs
    from basic research: An examination of the case of particle physics research. *CEPR
    Working Paper* 122 (January). Stanford, Calif.: Stanford University.

Financial Times. 1990. Making for the gaps left by giants. February 14, p. 16.

Florida, R., and Kenney, M. 1990. *The Breakthrough Illusion: Corporate America's
    Failure to Move From Innovation to Mass Production.* New York: Basic Books.

Gambardella, A. 1992. Competitive advantages from in-house basic research: The U.S.
    pharmaceutical industry in the 1980s. *Research Policy* 21:391–407.

Gambardella, A. 1995. Science and Innovation: The U.S. Pharmaceutical Industry in the
    1980s. Ph.D. thesis. Cambridge, Mass.: Cambridge University Press.

Grabowski, H. 1991. The changing economics of pharmaceutical research and develop-
    ment. In: Institute of Medicine. *Medical Innovation at the Crossroads*, vol. 2. *The
    Changing Economics of Medical Technology.* A. Gelijns and E. Halm, eds. Wash-
    ington, D.C.: National Academy Press, pp. 35–52.

Halperin, M., and Chakrabarti, A. 1987. Firm and industry characteristics influencing
    publications of scientists in large American companies. *R&D Management*
    17(3):169–173.

Imai, K. 1988. Japan's corporate networks. Paper prepared for the Minit-JPERC Confer-
    ence, Stanford University, Stanford, Calif., August 22–24, 1988.

Kenney, M. 1986. *Biotechnology: The University-Industry Complex.* New Haven,
    Conn.: Yale University Press.

Lerner, J. 1991. New biotechnology firms, capital markets, and innovation. Unpublished
    manuscript. Cambridge, Mass.: Department of Economics, Harvard University.

Merges, P., and Nelson, R. 1990. On the complex economics of patent scope. *Columbia
    Law Review* 90(4):840–916.

Mowery, D. C. 1981. The Emergence and Growth of Industrial Research in American
    Manufacturing 1899–1945. Ph.D. thesis. Stanford, Calif.: Stanford University.

Mowery, D. C., ed. 1988. *International Collaborative Ventures in U.S. Manufacturing.*
    Cambridge, Mass.: Ballinger Publishing Co.

Narin, F., et al. 1987. Patents as indicators of corporate technological strength. *Research
    Policy* 16:143–155.

Nelson, R. 1961. Uncertainty, learning, and the economics of parallel research and
    development efforts. *Review of Economics and Statistics* 43:351–364.

Office of Technology Assessment, U.S. Congress. 1984. *Commercial Biotechnology: An
    International Analysis.* OTA-BA-218. Washington, D.C.: U.S. Congress.

Orsenigo, L. 1989. *The Emergence of Biotechnology: Institutions and Markets in Indus-
    trial Innovation.* London: Francis Pinter.

Pisano, G. P. 1990. The R&D boundaries of the firm: An empirical analysis. *Adminis-
    trative Science Quarterly* 35:153–176.

Pisano, G. P., Shan, W., and Teece, D. J. 1988. Joint ventures and collaboration in the
    biotechnology industry. In: D. C. Mowery, ed. *International Collaborative Ven-
    tures in U.S. Manufacturing.* Cambridge, Mass.: Ballinger Publishing Co.

Rosenberg, N. 1990. Why do firms do basic research? *Research Policy* 19:165–174.

Scrip. 1991. Sandoz' biotech discovery initiative. March 20, p. 7.

Swann, J. P. 1988. *Academic Scientists and the Pharmaceutical Industry.* Baltimore, Md.: The John Hopkins University Press.

Telling, F. W. 1992. Managed care and pharmaceutical innovation. In: Institute of Medicine. 1992. *Medical Innovation at the Crossroads,* vol. 3. *Technology and Health Care in an Era of Limits.* A. C. Gelijns, ed. Washington, D.C.: National Academy Press.

Thackeray, A. 1982. University scientists in the chemical industry. In: National Science Board, ed. *University-Industry Research Relationships.* Washington, D.C.: U.S. Government Printing Office.

Thomas, L. G. 1988. Multifirm strategies in the U.S. pharmaceutical industry. In: D. C. Mowery, ed. *International Collaborative Ventures in U.S. Manufacturing.* Cambridge, Mass.: Ballinger Publishing Co.

Williamson, O. E. 1985. *The Economic Institutions of Capitalism.* New York: Free Press.

PART IV

Concluding Observations

9

Perspectives on Industrial R&D Management

GERALD D. LAUBACH

The case study approach to the examination of any issue always presents difficulties of extrapolation to the general from the particular. This is especially so as regards the inferences that might be drawn from the cases presented in this book that describe industrial research and development (R&D) directed to medical technology. There are two principal difficulties: first, the immense diversity of the industries that generate medical technology and, second, the drastic changes that are occurring in those industries as a consequence of the ongoing restructuring of American health care itself.

The principal industrial segments that develop and supply medical technology include large, generally multinational, pharmaceutical firms; the more than 1,000, mostly very small, venture-type firms that make up the biotechnology industry; both large and small firms that provide diagnostic tests and reagents; medical instrument divisions of large, diversified manufacturing firms; and the many, mostly smaller, specialized medical device firms. As will become apparent later in this chapter, two additional industries have become increasingly prominent influences upon medical technology—the large for-profit and not-for-profit "managed care" enterprises that now deliver more than half of the health care that Americans receive, and the host of systems-based firms that have sprung up to provide services of all kinds to the health care industry.

The firms encompassed in these diverse segments obviously differ greatly in sheer size and complexity, as well as in financial strength and stability. They vary also in the degree to which research and innovation is important to the overall success of the enterprise. One would surmise that an R&D project might be managed with more intensity, and more corporate oversight, in a biotechnol-

209

ogy venture whose very survival depends on research success, than would be the case for that same project embedded in a multibillion dollar corporation! One might also surmise that R&D projects with long time horizons, or much technical uncertainty, or foreseeable complexities in clinical or regulatory assessment, would be judged less feasible by a small, thinly financed firm than by a firm with ample resources. Industrial R&D management—its strategies, emphasis, direction—is influenced by the circumstances in which the firm finds itself—or perhaps more aptly, perceives itself—and all the forces at play may not be apparent to the author of a case study.

But the dramatic, recent changes in the structure of American health care represent one highly visible, and very potent, force that is impacting R&D in every sector of the health care technology industry. The earlier volumes of the *Medical Innovation at the Crossroads* series, beginning with the first in 1990, have documented, and in several cases anticipated, the effects of the changing health care market upon technology suppliers.

What are those changes? At considerable risk of oversimplification, of reiteration of the now obvious, and of gross disservice to the systematic analyses provided in chapters from earlier volumes of this series (for example, Soper and Ferris, 1992), I offer the following brief sketch:

Health care in America used to be a cottage industry. The adoption and use of health care technology were substantially under the control of several hundred thousand practicing physicians and surgeons. Those physicians and surgeons had strong professional motivations to adopt new technology; they also often had economic incentives to utilize technology.

The health care system that is emerging today has many of the characteristics of a true industrial enterprise. Acquisition of technology is controlled on the basis of its cost and value to the health care delivery firm. There is reluctance to accept technology that is new, or technology whose value has not been compellingly demonstrated. Large purchasers use their buying power to negotiate price. They require suppliers of similar technologies to bid against each other. They may exclude costly technologies altogether. They monitor, and attempt to control, the use of technology by the physicians and surgeons who are part of the enterprise.

THE CHANGING RESEARCH ENVIRONMENT

These changes in the market for health care technology are impacting industrial R&D in three principal ways: (1) they threaten established industry structure, modi operandi, and the financial resources of the technology suppliers; (2) they redefine the criteria for acceptability of new medical technologies; and (3) they impact the processes through which some technologies have historically been developed.

The symptoms of structural and financial stress in the industries that supply

TABLE 9-1 Major Acquisitions and Mergers of U.S. Pharmaceutical and Biotechnology Companies

Pharmaceutical Companies		Biotechnology Companies	
American Cyanamid and Immunex	1993	American Cyanamid and Immunex	1993
Procordia and Erbamont	1993	American Home and Genetics Institute	1991
Hoechst-Celanese (Hoechst) and Copley	1993	Boehringer Mannheim and Microgenics	1991
Marion Merrell Dow and generics		Sandoz and SyStemix	1991
operation of Rugby Darby	1993	Abbot and Damon Biotech	1990
Beecham and SmithKline	1991	Baxter and Bioresponce	1990
Boots and Flint	1990	Schering AG and Codon	1990
American Home and A. H. Robins	1989	Roche and Genentech	1990
Bristol-Myers and Squibb	1989	American Cyanamid and Praxis	1989
Dow and Marion	1989	Chugay and GenProbe	1989
Merck and DuPont	1989	Fujisawa and Lyphomed	1989
Merck and Johnson & Johnson	1989	Eli Lilly and Hybritech	1986
Kodak and Sterling	1988	Bristol-Myers and Genetic Systems	1985
Schering-Plough and Key	1986		
Monsanto and Searle	1986		
Rorer and USV/Armour	1986		
Rhône-Poulenc and Rorer	1983		

NOTE: The acquiror is noted first, and may be either a U.S. or a foreign company. The acquired company is noted second and is a U.S. company.

SOURCE: Adapted from the Boston Consulting Group, 1993, p. 42.

health care technology are now ubiquitous. Notable examples include the dramatic consolidation under way in the multinational pharmaceutical industry (a few of the major mergers and acquisitions are summarized in Table 9-1); the diversification of major pharmaceutical manufacturers into health care delivery, through acquisition of, or partnering with, firms that manage pharmacy benefits; consolidation (Table 9-1) and extensive partnering (Read and Lee, 1994) in the biotechnology industry; sharply depressed stock prices of pharmaceutical, biotechnology, and medical device firms for the past two years (Read and Lee, 1994); the reduced flow of new equity capital into the biotechnology and medical device industries (Littell, 1994; Read and Lee, 1994); and personnel cutbacks and downsizing reported by numerous firms in the health care technology industries.

Most of the changes related above are too recent to have had an observable effect on the level of R&D activity in the affected industries. Nonetheless, it seems unlikely that the consolidation of duplicate functions that normally accompanies the merger of similar firms will fail to impact research departments. Nor is it likely that firms in financial stress will neglect to scrutinize R&D budgets. Since virtually all of the capital raised by the smaller biotechnology and device firms is expended on R&D, the continued confidence of investors has a direct linkage to continuing research in those industries.

The criteria that the new health care marketplace establishes for acceptance of technology will define the targets for research in the health care technology firm. Since the market prizes cost-saving technology, R&D will seek to reduce the cost of existing technologies; will seek to replace costly technologies with more economical alternatives; and will carry out cost-effectiveness studies to make the economic case for the acceptance of their technologies. All of these phenomena are already evident (Gelijns and Rosenberg, 1994; Marshall, 1994; Telling, 1992). Since the market enforces price competition among similar technologies, research will target prospective new technologies that are meaningfully differentiated, that is, truly something new. Some existing technologies may enjoy longer lives than was typical heretofore, if the probability of finding substantially superior alternatives is judged to be low. The great attractiveness of highly differentiated—truly new—technologies will cause major emphasis to be given to applied research at the frontiers of basic science, with implications for the university-industry interface that are discussed further below.

Finally, some of the changes in the health care system interact with the R&D process itself. Here, unfortunately, the outlook is especially worrisome. The reasons are apparent in every one of the medical device and instrumentation cases detailed in earlier chapters. Those cases demonstrate lucidly two important characteristics of much medical innovation: first, that many truly revolutionary medical technologies are the end product of a long series of incremental refinements, sometimes beginning with a progenitor technology of marginal medical significance; second, that the actual process of innovation may involve a great deal of "tinkering at the bedside"—the process of developing the requisite skills, and learning the true potential of a new technology, through experience in actual clinical use.

These historically important modes of innovation are clearly threatened by policies that raise barriers to the diffusion of modest, incremental technological change, and by policies that seek to standardize medical practice. To paraphrase a prescient observation made at one of our earlier workshops, the biggest danger we may be facing is that of freezing in place the status quo (Neumann and Weinstein, 1991, p. 31).

At greatest risk from such policies are innovation in surgical procedures and in medical devices and instrumentation. However, even pharmaceuticals, products though they are of extensive and elaborate R&D programs, have found important new uses as a result of applications discovered after the product entered widespread use (Gelijns and Rosenberg, 1994; Laubach et al., 1992).

The emergence of these new constraints in the health care marketplace constitutes a central challenge to R&D management in the medical device and instrumentation industries. They underscore the importance of collaboration at the interface for these technologies—not only the interface between engineers in industry and research-minded physicians in universities, but the further interface with actively practicing physicians and surgeons. Although not explicitly discussed in this workshop, the management of medical device R&D is also being confronted by significantly increased Food and Drug Administration (FDA) regulatory requirements for medical devices (Merrill, 1994). Because the device industry comprises many smaller firms, the resiliency of the industry to respond effectively to the uncertainties of its new environment is a concern. The sixth workshop of the Committee on Technological Innovation in Medicine, carried out in collaboration with a committee of the National Academy of Engineering, explored these issues and others in depth (Gelijns et al., forthcoming).

THE EVOLVING SCIENCE BASE

The cases presented in earlier chapters illustrate that the science base underlying medical devices and instrumentation substantially resides in science-based industries outside of the medical field. The rate and direction of technological innovation in these "donor" industries must therefore influence technological innovation in the derived medical technologies. The great growth in information processing technologies, and the cutback in development of military hardware, are changes of the sort that are likely to impact future medical innovation.

What then can be said about the prospects for research and innovation in those industry segments—pharmaceuticals, vaccines, biotechnology, diagnostic tests and reagents—whose most important science base is modern biology? The economic constraints upon R&D, coupled with much more stringent criteria for innovative success, very likely will prove to be the most severe challenges these industries have ever faced. Research and development in these industries, if it is to be successful in the future, must devise richer sources of truly differentiated new technologies and must become more efficient in discovering, developing, and proving their value.

The single most important countervailing resource these industries bring to the search for differentiated products is the power of the new biology. In arguing thus, it is important to be clear about what is meant by the term "new biology." Because "biotechnology" and "the biotechnology industry" have become such prominent and well-known features of the popular culture, there is an understandable tendency to equate all of the new biology with recombinant DNA protein synthesis. Indeed, two of the cases in this book (Chapters 7 and 8) focus on that particular technology, undoubtedly because some of the earliest and most important medical products to emerge from the biotechnology industry were products of work with recombinant DNA.

That this view of the scope and power of the new biology is too narrow is well illustrated by an examination of the research objectives of the biotechnology industry today, as described in the prospectuses of the publicly owned firms. Even a cursory review reveals that research based on recombinant protein synthesis has been augmented by many other approaches. Today's more typical biotechnology project is predicated on the hypothesis that the function or dysfunction of one or another fundamental biomechanism may be of medical importance, then seeks ways to manipulate that mechanism to achieve medical benefits.

Biotechnology projects, in the mode just described, have in fact joined the mainstream of modern, rational pharmaceutical research. Perhaps the landmark case of this genre was the work of George Hitchings, Gertrude Elion, and their colleagues, who tenaciously pursued the idea that by systematically interfering with the then newly elucidated biochemical steps involved in nucleic acid biosynthesis, useful therapeutic agents could be found. Their faith was richly rewarded by the discovery of several new medicines—including the anticancer drug 6-mercaptopurine, the immune suppressant azathioprine, and the antibacterial trimethoprim, each the first of its kind—and by the Nobel Prize for Physiology or Medicine in 1988 (Elion, 1988; Hitchings, 1988; Melmon and Flowers, 1993).

Sir James Black was awarded his Nobel Prize for research that resulted in the discovery of the ß-adrenergic blocking drugs (a landmark advance in the therapy of cardiovascular disease) and the histamine H_2 antagonists (the first truly effective drugs for gastric and duodenal ulcer). In both cases, the research strategy exploited newly identified bioreceptors, whose selective inhibition proved to be a successful pathway to a new class of medicines (Black, 1988).

In fact, a large proportion of the most significant pharmaceuticals introduced in recent years are products of research that took its departure from one or another fundamental insight into the intimate nature of a biological process (Laubach, 1983, 1994). Such is also the case for most of the newer chemical and immunological diagnostic tests.

The implications for the future of applied medical research are clear. The molecular workings of important biological processes are being elucidated at an astonishing rate. Literally dozens of genes, receptors, and mediators that play roles in controlling biological function have been discovered. In many cases, their significance, in normal function and in disease, is yet to be fully explored. This vast and rapidly expanding science base will undoubtedly be the launching pad for much applied medical research for years to come. However, this richness of opportunity is two-edged. It will demand great discrimination on the part of the R&D manager in selecting which biological pathway to pursue, and decisiveness in abandoning approaches that peter out.

The critical importance of the university-industry interface in R&D of this kind should also be clear. The patterns of interaction will doubtless continue to involve formal partnering arrangements mediated through biotechnology firms, as detailed in chapter 8 of this volume by Arora and Gambardella. At the other pole, they will merely involve the interplay of applied and basic research mediated through the scientific literature, the kind of open process well illustrated by the work of Hitchings, Elion and Black and, indeed, by most of the modern therapeutic agents that have clearly discernible roots in basic science. But whatever the pattern of interaction at the interface, bridging the culture gap between academic and industrial science will doubtless remain a nontrivial challenge for R&D management.

Techniques and methodologies emerging from the new biology are also germane to the pressing need to increase the efficiency of the discovery process. A number of firms in the pharmaceutical and biotechnology industries have focused on the development of technologies that allow the rapid, automated synthesis of thousands, or even millions, of experimental substances for preliminary screening ("combinatorial chemistry"). Counterpart technologies have been developed that allow massive, "parallel processing" exposure of such chemical libraries to biological test systems (receptor molecules in vitro, for example) to expedite the first steps in selecting prospective therapeutic leads (for example, see Gallop et al., 1994; Gordon et al., 1994). A variety of other prospectively powerful research approaches are being explored—gene therapy is one—that, if successful, promise virtually direct translation of basic research findings into therapeutic applications (Schwartz, 1994).

CLINICAL EVALUATION OF NEW TECHNOLOGIES

The efficiency of the *development* process for therapeutic technologies based on biology represents a separate and significant issue in R&D management. The lion's share of the money and time required by the R&D process leading to a new pharmaceutical is dedicated to clinical trials to demonstrate safety and efficacy. The new kinds of therapeutic modalities likely to emerge from research of the sorts just described may well pose challenging new problems in clinical evaluation. Market demands for the demonstration of cost-effectiveness, impact on patient quality of life, and relative value versus other therapeutic modalities can only increase the complexity and cost of clinical trials. Clearly, a major challenge to R&D management lies at the interface with the evaluative clinical sciences.

The very first workshop of the *Medical Innovation at the Crossroads* series was devoted to an exploration of newer methods of clinical evaluation, including an examination of their potential for facilitating the evaluation of medical technologies of all kinds (Institute of Medicine, 1990). Many of these methodologies are being put to good use. But the most intriguing opportunity may prove to lie in a reexamination of how we define the interface between experimental and established medical technology.

This is currently an unsettled matter, involving substantial dissatisfaction and no little confusion. Witness, for example, the controversies surrounding the so-called "early release" of AIDS drugs by the FDA, or the controversies and litigation over reimbursement of experimental cancer therapies (see, for instance,

Institute of Medicine, 1994, for discussion of the latter). The path to resolution of the question is not clear, although both public and private providers of health care are exploring options (Reiser, 1994).

In principle at least, one particularly provocative option is suggested by the quasi-industrial structure that is emerging in American health care delivery. Other technology-dependent industries commonly do substantial in-house research, including collaboration with their technology suppliers in the evaluation and in-transfer of new technologies. Such activities offer economic benefits, by providing more timely and efficient adaptation of a new technology to the specific needs of the user firm. They also can constitute an effective mode of interfirm competition.

Large health care delivery firms, with their vast data bases and captive patient populations, are excellently positioned to undertake evaluative research on medical technologies, and some of them are increasingly doing so. Since much present-day medical technology is both costly and limited in its effectiveness, health care providers in today's competitive environment should be strongly motivated to be leaders in seeking out, and adopting, superior technologies. As such practices mature, they may well modulate the notion that there is, and should be, a single, one-size-fits-all transition between the experimental and the established medical technology.

CONCLUDING OBSERVATIONS

The interaction between industrial suppliers of health care technology and the industrial providers of health care services is clearly an important feature in the changing landscape of American medicine. These changes are impacting the resources available for research toward new medical technology, its direction, and even the ways it is carried out. The traditionally important interface between industrial R&D and universities will remain, and even grow in importance. But the interface between industrial R&D and the industrial providers of health care may well prove to be the most critical interface of all for the industrial R&D managers of tomorrow.

REFERENCES

Black, J. 1988. Drugs from emasculated hormones: The principles of syntopic antagonism. In J. Hindsten, ed. 1993. *Nobel Lectures, Physiology or Medicine 1981–1990*. World Scientific Press: River Edge, N.J., pp. 418–440.

Boston Consulting Group. 1993. *The Changing Environment for U.S. Pharmaceuticals: The Role of Pharmaceutical Companies in a Systems Approach to Health Care.* Boston Consulting Group: Boston, Mass.

Elion, G. B. 1988. The purine path to chemotherapy. In J. Hindsten, ed. 1993. *Nobel*

Lectures, Physiology or Medicine 1981–1990. World Scientific Press: River Edge, N.J., pp. 447–468.

Gallop, M. A., Barrett, R. W., Dower, W. J., et al. 1994. Applications of combinatorial technologies to drug discovery. 1. Background and peptide combinatorial liberaries. *Journal of Medical Chemistry* 37:1233–1251.

Gelijns, A. C. and Rosenberg, N. 1994. The dynamics of technological change in medicine. *Health Affairs* 13(3):28–46.

Gordon, E. M., Barrett, R. W., Dower, W. J., et al. 1994. Applications of combinatorial technologies to drug discovery. 2. Combinational organic synthesis, library screening strategies, and future directions. *Journal of Medical Chemistry* 37:1385–1401.

Hitchings, G. 1988. Selective inhibitors of dehydrofolate reductase. In J. Hindsten, ed. 1993. *Nobel Lectures, Physiology or Medicine 1981–1990.* World Scientific Press: River Edge, N.J., pp. 476–493.

Institute of Medicine. 1990. *Medical Innovation at the Crossroads,* vol. 1. *Modern Methods of Clinical Investigation.* A. C. Gelijns, ed. Washington, D.C.: National Academy Press.

Institute of Medicine. 1994. *Medical Innovation at the Crossroads,* vol. 4. *Adopting New Medical Technology.* A. C. Gelijns and H. V. Dawkins, eds. Washington, D.C.: National Academy Press.

Laubach, G. D. 1983. The chemical basis for modern therapeutics. *The Chemist* 60(1):6,18–19.

Laubach, G. D. 1994. Perspective. Growing pains: A more optimistic view. *Health Affairs* 13(3):194–196.

Laubach, G. D., Wennberg, J. E., and Gelijns, A. C. 1992. In: Institute of Medicine. *Medical Innovation at the Crossroads,* vol. 3. *Technology and Health Care in an Era of Limits.* A. C. Gelijns, ed. Washington, D.C.: National Academy Press, pp. 3–8.

Littell, C. L. 1994. Datawatch. Innovation in medical technology: Reading the indicators. *Health Affairs* 13(3):226–235.

Marshall, A. K. M. 1994. Manufacturers' responses to the increased demand for outcomes research. In: Institute of Medicine. *Medical Innovation at the Crossroads,* vol. 3. *Technology and Health Care in an Era of Limits.* A. C. Gelijns and H. V. Dawkins, eds. Washington, D.C.: National Academy Press, pp. 152–171.

Melmon, K., and Flowers, C. 1993. Purine metabolism and the development of chemotherapeutic agents. Unpublished paper, Stanford University.

Merrill, R. A. 1994. Regulation of drugs and devices: An evolution. *Health Affairs* 13(3):47–69.

Neumann, P. J., and Weinstein, M. C. 1991. The diffusion of new technology: Costs and benefits to health care. In: Institute of Medicine. *Medical Innovation at the Crossroads,* vol. 2. *The Changing Economics of Medical Technology.* A. C. Gelijns and E. A. Halm, eds. Washington, D.C.: National Academy Press, pp. 21–34.

Read, J. L., and Lee, K. B., Jr. 1994. Datawatch. Health care innovation: Progress report and focus on biotechnology. *Health Affairs* 13(3):215–225.

Reiser, S. J. 1994. Criteria for standard versus experimental therapy. *Health Affairs* 13(3):127–136.

Schwartz, W. B. 1994. In the pipeline: A wave of valuable medical technology. *Health Affairs* 13(3):70–79.

Soper, M., and Ferris, D. 1992. The growth of managed care in the private sector. In: Institute of Medicine. *Medical Innovation at the Crossroads*, vol. 3. *Technology and Health Care in an Era of Limits*. A. C. Gelijns, ed. Washington, D.C.: National Academy Press, pp. 37–50.

Telling, F. V. 1992. Managed care and pharmaceutical innovation. In: Institute of Medicine. *Medical Innovation at the Crossroads*, vol. 3. *Technology and Health Care in an Era of Limits*. A. C. Gelijns, ed. Washington, D.C.: National Academy Press, pp. 201–218.

10

The Intertwining of Public and Proprietary in Medical Technology

RICHARD R. NELSON

As I reflect on the papers presented at the fifth workshop in the series *Medical Innovation at the Crossroads*, and on the discussion, I am struck by how little was said about a topic my instincts tell me is of large and increasing importance: the intertwining of public and proprietary in medical technology, and the actual and potential conflicts associated with that intertwining.

In virtually all of the histories of medical innovation presented at the workshop, both universities and firms were involved at various stages. Both public and private monies contributed to the development of the technology. The findings of the research and the news of the new techniques were published in scientific papers and spread across the community of relevant professionals through talks and discussions at scientific and professional society meetings, and also through informal communication. At the same time, in many cases patents were filed for and granted at particular stages of the process.

There is a myth that is widely held among scholars, as well as among lay persons, that "science" and "technology" define two quite separate as well as different cultures. Science is what academics do, and scientists openly publish and otherwise communicate their findings. Technology is what business firms or profit-oriented private inventors do, and they patent their successes. There is a related myth that the relationship between science and technology is one where technologists draw freely on public science that was created with no notion at all as to its likely uses in the development of technology. The problem with these two myths is that they are largely myths. In fact, the worlds of science and technology are, in many fields, closely intertwined. Much of "science" is done with the express purpose of illuminating various areas of possible "technology" development. People at universities develop new technologies, and people at firms do publish new science. The intertwining of science and technology is particularly prevalent, it seems to me, in the arena of medical research and innovation.

The advent of modern biotechnology certainly has exacerbated the intertwining problem, but the intertwining has been there for a long time. Consider, for example, the intertwining of science and technology, and universities and industry, in the development of purified insulin. The tradition of American patent law rules out the patenting of "natural substances" or "scientific principles." However, purified natural substances have been patentable, and several of the key patents in biotechnology come pretty close to being on "scientific principles." The recent argument and uproar about patenting gene fragments has quieted down for a while, but that issue will not go away. Nor will the debate about whether companies who patent new substances that draw extensively on government-financed public science, such as zidovudine (AZT), should be free to charge any price that they like. A recent issue of *Science* reported on the uproar that was caused when some university researchers doing sleep research filed for a patent on a particular technique that their colleagues claimed was part of general knowledge among those working at the frontier in that field.

It seems to me that there are two important sets of questions here. The first is: What is public and what in fact is proprietary, and what are the factors that make for the present divide? It is obvious, for example, that the use of patents differs widely across three different fields of medical technology—pharmaceuticals, medical devices, and medical techniques and practices—with patents playing an important role in the first, and hardly any role at all in the last. (This is certainly one of the reasons why the filing noted above for a patent on a technique caused such an uproar.) However, the reasons for these differences are not entirely clear, nor are their consequences in terms of the nature of the research and inventing work done by different parties. The latter issue leads naturally to the second set of questions: What *should* be kept public and what should be allowed to be proprietary? Patent law and practice is made, and remade, by Congress and the courts. Both Congress and the courts have shown themselves to be relatively responsive to professional opinions. The issue of patenting the human genome is a dramatic instance, but only one of many, where the question of what should be patentable and what should not began to be discussed.

While I will not develop these issues further here, it seems to me that regarding the latter set of questions there are three matters that deserve a lot more attention than they currently have received. One is the increasing tendency of the Patent Office and the courts to allow and uphold patents on what might well be regarded as "scientific findings." A second matter is that neither the Patent Office nor the courts at present have any way of tapping into what professionals in a field already know, unless there is a written and published articulation of knowledge. Third, I think the time is ripe for a reconsideration of the question of private ownership rights to patents that come out of publicly funded research.

APPENDIXES

APPENDIX A

Workshop Agenda

THE UNIVERSITY-INDUSTRY INTERFACE
AND MEDICAL INNOVATION

Sunday, February 21, 1993

2:30 p.m.   **Welcome**
             Kenneth Shine, President, Institute of Medicine

             Introduction to the Workshop
             Enriqueta Bond, Executive Officer, Institute of Medicine

SESSION I. SETTING THE STAGE

Moderator: Ken Melmon, Stanford University
             Some Further Thoughts on the Origin of the Workshop

3:00   **Medical Innovation and the Economic Environment**
             Victor Fuchs, Stanford University

3:30   **R&D Management: An Academic Perspective**
             Stanley Cohen, Stanford University

4:00   **Institutional Factors Affecting the University-Industry Interface**
             Niels Reimers, Technology Linkages International

4:30   Discussion

5:00   **R&D Management: An Industrial Perspective**
              Alejandro Zaffaroni, ALZA Corporation

5:30   **The Evolution of Biotechnology Drugs at AMGEN and ICOS**
              George Rathmann, ICOS

Respondent: Joel Birnbaum, Hewlett-Packard

6:00   Discussion

7:00   Adjourn and Dinner

Monday, February 22, 1993

8:15 a.m.   Continental Breakfast

SESSION II. MEDICAL DEVICE INNOVATION

Moderator: Bill Hubbard, Former President, The Upjohn Company

Respondents: Ben Holmes, Hewlett-Packard; James Benson, Health Industry
              Manufacturers Association; and Harvey Rudolph, Food and Drug
              Administration

8:45   **Minimally Invasive Therapy: The Case of Endoscopy**
              Introduction: Nathan Rosenberg, Stanford University, and
              Annetine Gelijns, Institute of Medicine/Columbia University
              Discussion

9:45   **The Laser in Medicine: Birth of a New Industry**
              Introduction: Joanne Spetz, Stanford University
              Discussion

10:45   Break

11:00   **Cardiovascular Diagnostics**
              Introduction: Stan Finkelstein, Massachusetts Institute of
              Technology, Gregory Bell, Charles River Associates, and
              Kevin Neels, Quintiles
              Discussion

12:00   **Medical Imaging: MRI and PET**
Introduction: Richard Rettig, Institute of Medicine, Holly
Dawkins, Institute of Medicine, and Everette James, Vanderbilt
University
Discussion

1:00   Lunch

2:15   **Cochlear Implants**
Introduction: Stuart Blume, University of Amsterdam
Discussion

SESSION III. PHARMACEUTICAL AND BIOTECH INNOVATION

Moderator: Stanley Reiser, University of Texas Health Science Center

Respondents: Gerald Laubach, Former President, Pfizer; Rebecca Henderson,
Massachusetts Institute of Technology; James Benson, Health
Industry Manufacturers Association

3:15   **Purine Metabolism and the Development of Chemotherapeutic Agents**
Introduction: Chris Flowers and Ken Melmon, Stanford
University
Discussion

4:15   Break

4:30   **Innovation in Biotechnology: The Case of the Small Firm**
Introduction: Alfonso Gambardella, Bocconi University, Milan,
and Ashish Arora, Carnegie-Mellon University
Discussion

5:30   Adjournment

Tuesday, February 23, 1993

SESSION III. PHARMACEUTICAL AND BIOTECH INNOVATION
(continued)

Moderator: Stanley Reiser, University of Texas Health Science Center

Respondents: Gerald Laubach, Former President, Pfizer; Rebecca Henderson,
              Massachusetts Institute of Technology; James Benson, Health
              Industry Manufacturers Association

8:00 a.m.   **Innovation in Compounds to Treat Diabetes**
              Introduction: Scott Stern, Stanford University
              Discussion

9:00   **What Is Public? What Is Private? And What Should Be?**
              Richard Nelson, Columbia University
              Discussion

9:30   General Discussion

10:00   Break

10:30   **Where Do We Go From Here?**
              Ken Melmon, Stanford University
              Richard Nelson, Columbia University
              Nathan Rosenberg, Stanford University

11:00   Adjournment

APPENDIX B

Contributors

ASHISH ARORA is assistant professor of economics at the H. John Heinz School of Public Policy at Carnegie-Mellon University. He has a Ph.D. in economics from Stanford University. His research focuses on the economics of technological change, intellectual property rights and technology licensing, technology transfer to developing countries, and the patterns of specialization and division of labor in industrial structure. Recently Dr. Arora co-authored a report to the National Institute of Standards and Technology on Manufacturing Technology Centers. He is currently a visiting scholar at Stanford University, carrying out research on the dynamics of international comparative advantage in the chemical industry.

GREGORY K. BELL is senior associate at Charles River Associates (CRA) and heads their health economics consulting practice. He specializes in business and marketing strategy for the health-related industry. He has played a key role in a variety of projects dealing with international investment policy, pricing strategy, transfer pricing, OTC switches, and management of R&D process. In the health technology area, Dr. Bell works with firms to develop sustainable competitive advantages in specific product markets. Before joining CRA, Dr. Bell taught at Harvard University, developing and leading a course on the economics of business strategy. He received his Ph.D. in business economics from Harvard University and his M.B.A. from the Harvard Graduate School of Business Administration.

STUART BLUME has been professor and chair of the Department of Science and Technology Dynamics, University of Amsterdam, The Netherlands, since 1982. Between 1977 and 1980 he was research secretary of the Committee on Social Inequalities in Health, Department of Health and Social Security, London. Since that time, his research has focused in particular on sociological aspects of medical research and innovation. Principal publications in this area include *Insight and Industry: The Dynamics of Technological Change in Medicine* (MIT Press, 1992); (with A. Hiddinga) "Social contexts of technological change in medicine: The origins and transformation of obstetric pelvimetry" in *Science, Technology and Human Values* (1992); and "Social process and the assessment of a new imaging technique" in the *International Journal of Technology Assessment in Health Care* (1993). Dr. Blume has been a consultant to the OECD for many years and was recently president of the Research Committee on Sociology of Science of the International Sociological Association.

ENRIQUETA C. BOND is president of the Burroughs Wellcome Fund, a private independent foundation with a mission to advance the medical sciences. Her past employment experiences have included the position of executive director of the Institute of Medicine and faculty positions at Southern Illinois University School of Medicine and at Chatham College. She has a B.A. from Wellesley College in zoology and physiology, an M.A. in genetics from the University of Virginia, and a Ph.D. in molecular biology from Georgetown University.

HOLLY V. DAWKINS is a research assistant in the Divisions of Health Care at the Institute of Medicine. Since joining the Institute of Medicine in June 1988, she has worked on over a dozen IOM projects, in particular the IOM program on technological innovation in medicine and the series *Medical Innovation at the Crossroads*. In 1991, she received the Institute of Medicine staff award for her work on the Institute of Medicine study to evaluate the artificial heart program of the National Heart, Lung, and Blood Institute. Holly earned her A.B. with honors in English from Brown University in 1986.

STAN N. FINKELSTEIN is senior lecturer in Health Policy and Management at the Massachusetts Institute of Technology (MIT) Sloan School of Management and a consultant for Charles River Associates. He received the S.M. and S.B. degrees from MIT in chemical engineering in 1971 and the M.D. from Harvard Medical School in 1975. Since 1975, he has actively worked in the field of medical technology assessment and transfer at MIT where he has conducted research and taught classes in the areas of the development and evaluation of medical practice and technology and in health policy. Among his interests have been the business-government interface related to the pharmaceutical industry, especially clinical research design and third party reimbursement. Dr. Finkelstein is author, editor, or contributor to books and numerous articles on these subjects.

ALFONSO GAMBARDELLA received his Ph.D. in economics from Stanford University in 1990. He is currently associate professor at the University of Urbino, and senior research fellow at Bocconi University, Milano, in Italy. He has carried out research on the relationship between science and the innovation process and in the areas of the management of the R&D process. He is currently working on the economics of scientific institutions, examining the factors that influence the nature and efficiency of university-based research. Dr. Gambardella has recently published a book (Cambridge University Press) on corporate strategies in R&D in the pharmaceutical industry.

ANNETINE C. GELIJNS is director of the International Center on Health Outcomes and Innovation Research, and an assistant professor in the Department of Surgery, College of Physicians and Surgeons, and the School of Public Health, Columbia University, New York City. Her current research focuses on the factors driving the rate and direction of innovative activity in medicine, technological change and its relation to health care costs, and measuring the outcomes of surgical care. Before coming to Columbia in 1993, she directed the Program on Technological Innovation in Medicine at the Institute of Medicine, National Academy of Sciences. From 1983–1987, she worked for the Steering Committee on Future Health Scenarios and for the Health Council, the Netherlands. Dr. Gelijns has been a consultant to various national and international organizations, including the World Health Organization and the Organization for Economic Cooperation and Development. She holds a Ph.D. from the medical faculty, University of Amsterdam, and bachelors and masters degrees in law from the University of Leyden, the Netherlands.

SIMON GLYNN received his B.A. degree from Wesleyan University in 1990 and currently is involved in projects for the Institute of Medicine, as well as the National Academy of Engineering (NAE). Prior to starting at the Institute of Medicine he was senior analyst at Gemini Consulting.

GERALD D. LAUBACH holds a B.A. from the University of Pennsylvania and a Ph.D. in organic chemistry from the Massachusetts Institute of Technology. He was formerly president of Pfizer, Inc., and is the chair of the IOM Committee on Technological Innovation in Medicine. Dr. Laubach is a research chemist by training and served as a laboratory scientist in his early years at Pfizer. He is a member of the Institute of Medicine and the National Academy of Engineering, and served on the now disbanded IOM Council on Health Care Technology. His current activities also include membership on the executive committee of the Council on Competitiveness (successor group to the President's Commission on

Industrial Competitiveness), the board of the Food and Drug Law Institute, the Corporation of the Rockefeller University Council, the Carnegie Institution of Washington, the National Committee for Quality Health Care, the Medical Center Advisory Board, the New York Hospital–Cornell Medical Center, and the Corporation Committee for Sponsored Research at the Massachusetts Institute of Technology; he is a director of CIGNA Corporation of Philadelphia and the Millpore Corporation of Bedford, Massachusetts. Previously, Dr. Laubach served as chair of the Pharmaceutical Manufacturers Association from 1977 to 1978 and as a board member until April 1989. He has received honorary doctorates in humane letters from the City University of New York, in law from Connecticut College, and in science from Hofstra University.

KEVIN NEELS is vice president, health economics, at Quintiles, Inc. Previously he served as vice president at Charles River Associates. He has played a key role in a wide range of projects dealing with questions of comparative effectiveness of medical therapies, impacts of public policy initiatives, and business strategy development. Previously, Dr. Neels worked at the Rand Corporation and the Urban Institute. He has authored numerous articles on housing and transportation and has offered expert testimony to the federal courts on the economic implications of alternative healthcare delivery arrangements. He received the bachelors, masters, and doctoral degrees from Cornell University.

RICHARD NELSON is the George Blumenthal Professor of International and Public Affairs, Business and Law, at Columbia University. Before coming to Columbia in 1986, he was professor of economics and director of the Institute for Social and Policy Studies at Yale University. He has served on the staff of the President's Council of Economic Advisors and has been involved in many activities concerned with molding better national policies. His central research interests have been economic growth; that interest has led him into a long career of study of technical advances and the institutions supporting and molding the processes involved. His most recent large project on these topics is described in the book *National Innovation Systems: A Comparative Analysis*, published in 1993 by the Oxford University Press.

NATHAN ROSENBERG is chair of the Department of Economics and professor of economics at Stanford University. Before assuming his current position, he served as chair of the Stanford Program on Values, Technology, and Society and as director of the Stanford Program on Public Policy. Dr. Rosenberg moved to Stanford in 1974; prior to that, he served on the faculties of the University of Wisconsin, Harvard University, Purdue University, and the University of Pennsylvania. He was a Fulbright Scholar at Queens' College, Oxford University, between 1952 and 1954 and a visiting Rockefeller Professor at the University of the Philippines in 1970 and 1971. Dr. Rosenberg served as editor of the *Journal* *of Economic History* between 1972 and 1974, and in 1981 he became a fellow of the American Academy of Arts and Sciences. Dr. Rosenberg is the author of numerous articles and several books, focusing for the most part on the history of technological change in industry. His most recent book, *Exploring the Black Box*, was published by Cambridge University Press in 1994. Dr. Rosenberg earned his B.A. degree from Rutgers University and his M.A. and Ph.D. degrees from the University of Wisconsin.

JOANNE SPETZ is a doctoral candidate in the Department of Economics at Stanford University. Her research interests include labor markets, medical technology, and hospital behavior. While at Stanford, she has been a National Science Foundation fellow and a recipient of a Bradley Foundation Fellowship. She is also a health research specialist at the Veterans' Administration Medical Center in Palo Alto. She completed her S.B. in economics at the Massachusetts Institute of Technology in 1990, received her M.A. in economics at Stanford University in 1993, and expects to complete her Ph.D. in 1995.

SCOTT STERN is completing his doctoral degree in economics at Stanford University. His dissertation focuses on the effects of competition and the management of innovation within pharmaceutical markets. He received his B.A. in economics from New York University in 1990.

Index